A Comprehensive Guide to Holistic Beauty

Discovering the Secrets of Natural Hair and Skincare

BY

Jenny Kings

Copyright 2023 Jenny Kings

License Notes

No part of this Book can be reproduced in any form or by any means including print, electronic, scanning or photocopying unless prior permission is granted by the author.

All ideas, suggestions and guidelines mentioned here are written for informative purposes. While the author has taken every possible step to ensure accuracy, all readers are advised to follow information at their own risk. The author cannot be held responsible for personal and/or commercial damages in case of misinterpreting and misunderstanding any part of this Book

Table of Contents

Introduction

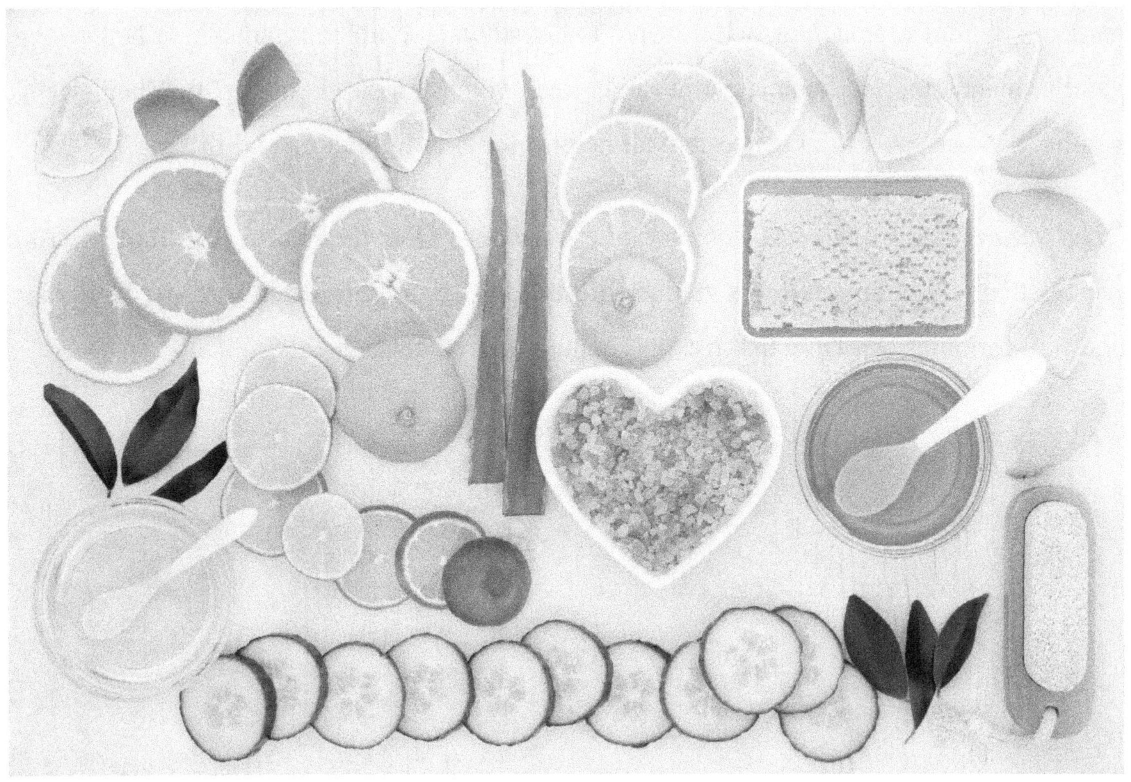

The green lifestyle is frequently touted for its supposed health benefits and low environmental impact. Each person who opts for natural and homemade remedies does so for their own unique reasons. The accumulation of chemicals in conventional cosmetic products is a major contributor. Sustainable, cruelty-free, and environmentally friendly natural cosmetic products are preferred by some. Many commercially available cosmetics pose serious risks to users' health. Toners, foundations, mascaras, moisturizers, cleansers, and lipstick are all items that women use often. Sixty percent of these cosmetics are absorbed by the skin.

Going green may help you avoid health problems and save you money on expensive cosmetics. You may color your hair with henna or any natural product. You can use mild components like oatmeal, lavender, mint, camomile, mango, grapefruit, calendula, gardenia, burdock, aloe vera, and coconut to get silky, smooth hair and skin. Ylang-ylang, vanilla, mandarin, and banana can all help keep your skin supple and soft. Ylang-ylang, vanilla, bananas, and strawberries are all helpful for skin tightening and firming.

"The Natural Beauty Bible: A Comprehensive Guide to Holistic Beauty" is full of fantastic recipes that will help you live a greener lifestyle. There are 30 different body, face, hair, and skin formulas available that use only natural ingredients.

OOOOOOOOOOOOOOOOOO

Chemical-Free Skin Peeling Treatments

The technique of peeling is well-known for its efficacy in removing dead skin cells and cleaning debris and oil from skin pores. The many chemicals used to peel the skin are harsh and out of reach for most individuals. There are a variety of natural options for improving skin health and appearance. Quickly and easily revive your skin with a homemade mask or tonic made from fresh fruits and vegetables. I'll be talking about some healthy ways to speed up your skin's natural peeling process, so you won't have to resort to dangerous and expensive products.

OOOOOOOOOOOOOOOOO

1. Cornstarch and Carrot Juice

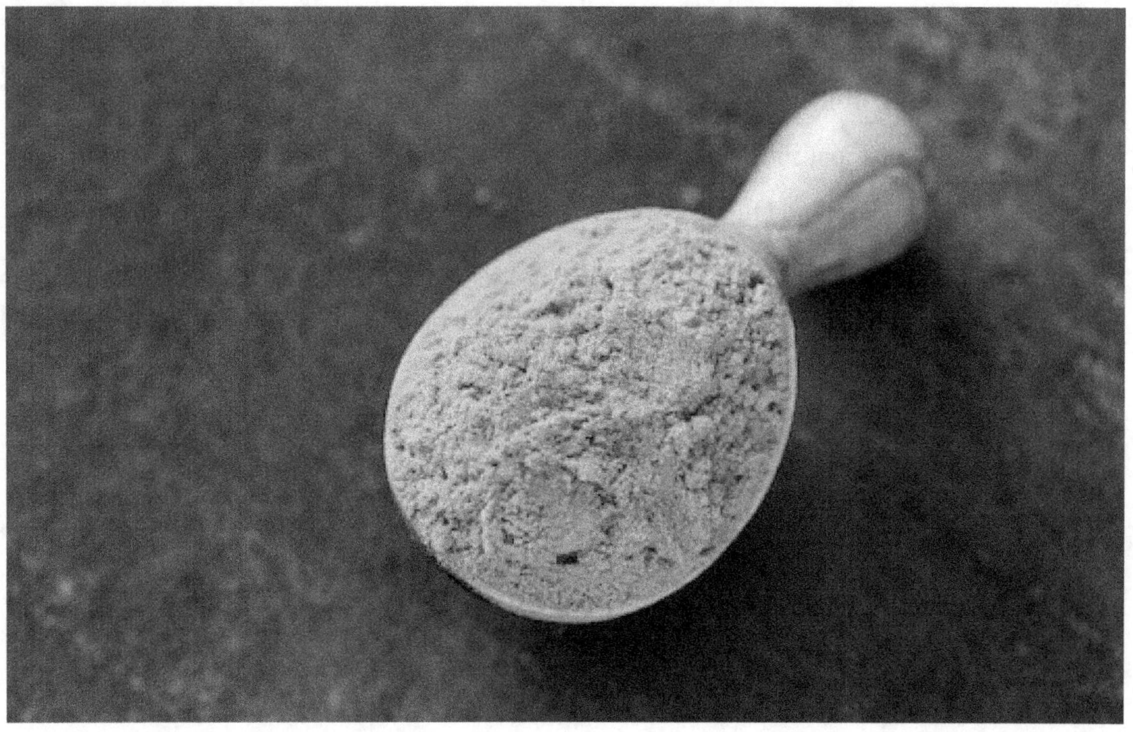

It is a soothing treatment to remove dead skin layers from your face.

Cooking Time: 5 minutes

Application Time: 15 minutes

List of Ingredients:

- Egg white: 1
- Carrot juice: 3 tablespoons
- Turmeric Powder: 1 teaspoon
- Cornstarch: 3 tablespoons

OOOOOOOOOOOOOOOOOO

Procedure:

A. In a bowl, stir together 3 tablespoons of cornstarch, 1 egg white, 1 teaspoon of turmeric powder, and 3 tablespoons of carrot juice. You can also blend the ingredients to achieve a smooth and fine paste.

B. Prior to applying the paste, cleanse your face thoroughly using a face wash or mild soap. Ensure that your face is clean and free from any makeup or impurities.

C. Using a soft brush or your fingers, apply the paste evenly onto your face. Avoid the delicate area around your eyes and lips.

D. Allow the paste to work on your skin for a duration of fifteen minutes. During this time, you may experience a tightening sensation as the ingredients work their magic.

E. After fifteen minutes, gently rinse your face with lukewarm water. Use a soft sponge or your hands to remove the paste thoroughly.

F. Pat your face dry with a clean towel. Avoid rubbing your skin harshly, as this may cause irritation.

G. Follow up with your regular skincare routine, such as applying moisturizer or any other skincare products you prefer. It is recommended to perform this treatment once or twice a week for optimal results.

Notes:

A. Turmeric powder may leave a slight yellow tint on your skin, but it will fade gradually.

B. If you have any known allergies or sensitivities to the ingredients, it is advisable to perform a patch test on a small area of your skin before applying the paste to your entire face.

C. This homemade chemical peel is suitable for most skin types, but if you have sensitive skin, it's essential to monitor your skin's reaction and adjust the ingredients accordingly.

D. Remember to protect your clothing and surroundings as turmeric powder may stain.

2. Artichoke and Vinegar

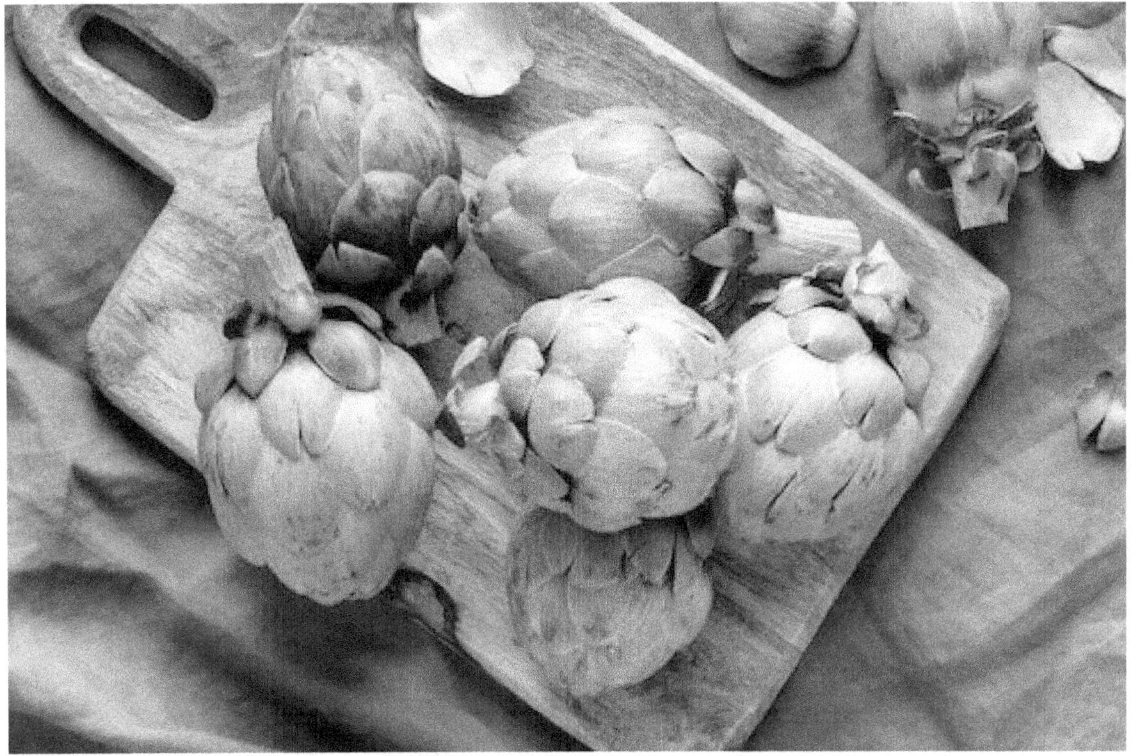

It is the best remedy to get deep cleansing treatments and to remove your dead skin cells.

Cooking Time: 5 minutes

Application Time: 15 minutes

List of Ingredients:

- Olive oil: 2 tablespoons
- Vinegar: 1 tablespoon
- Cooked Artichoke heart: 1

OOOOOOOOOOOOOOOOOO

Procedure:

A. Start by mashing a cooked artichoke heart using a fork or a food processor. Ensure that it is well-mashed to create a smooth texture.

B. In a small bowl, combine the mashed artichoke with 2 tablespoons of olive oil and 1 tablespoon of vinegar. Mix well to create a paste-like consistency.

C. Before applying the paste, cleanse your face using a gentle face wash or mild soap. Ensure that your face is free from any makeup or dirt.

D. With clean hands, gently massage the artichoke paste onto your face using circular motions. Pay attention to areas that may require extra attention, such as the forehead, nose, and cheeks.

E. Allow the paste to sit on your skin for a duration of 20 minutes. During this time, you may feel a tightening sensation as the ingredients work their magic.

F. After 20 minutes, take a clean washcloth and soak it in lukewarm water. Use the damp washcloth to gently wipe off the artichoke paste from your skin. Make sure to be gentle and avoid scrubbing too harshly.

G. Rinse your face with cool water to remove any remaining residue from the paste. Pat your skin dry with a clean towel.

A. This artichoke and vinegar peel is known for its exfoliating properties, helping to remove dead skin cells and leaving your skin refreshed.

B. If you have any known allergies or sensitivities to the ingredients, it is advisable to perform a patch test on a small area of your skin before applying the paste to your entire face.

C. This homemade chemical peel is suitable for most skin types, but if you have sensitive skin, it's essential to monitor your skin's reaction and adjust the ingredients accordingly.

D. Follow up with your regular skincare routine, such as applying moisturizer or any other skincare products you prefer.

E. It is recommended to perform this treatment once a week for best results.

3. Tomato and Cucumber

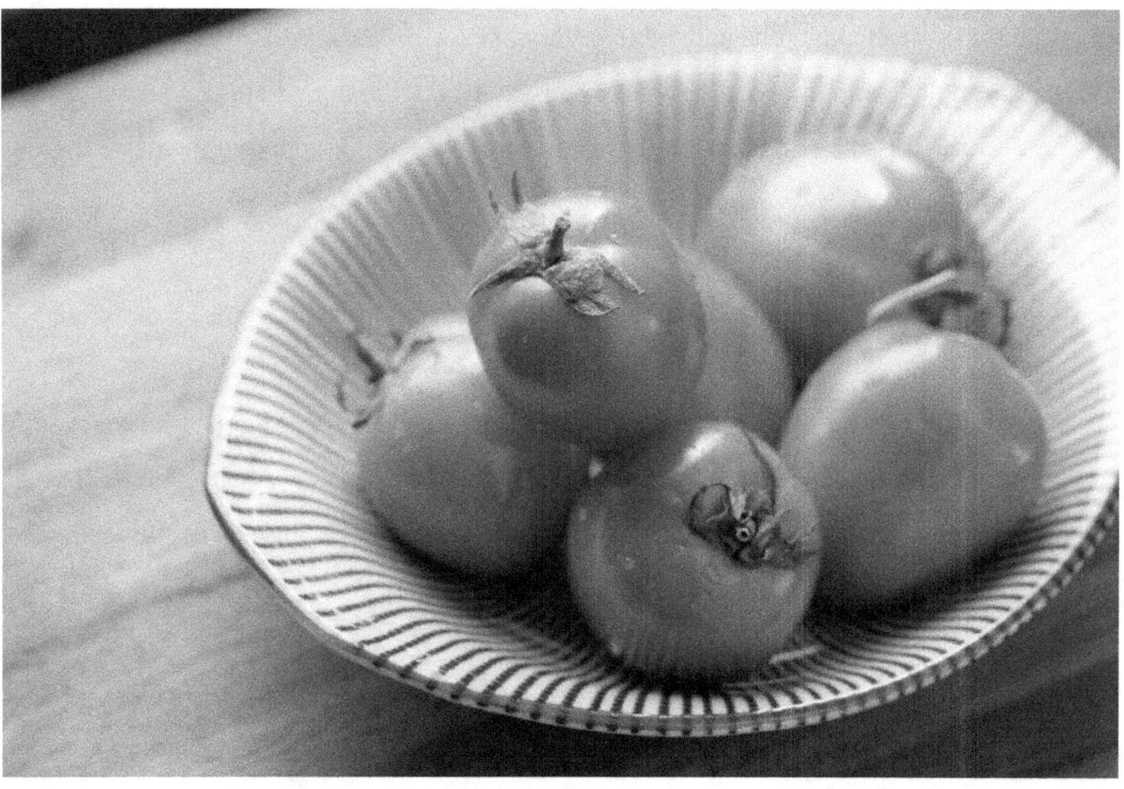

These both are perfect natural ingredients to purify your skin.

Cooking Time: 5 minutes

Application Time: 10 minutes

List of Ingredients:

- Mint leaves: 4
- Oatmeal: 3 tablespoons
- Sour milk: 2 teaspoons
- Crushed cucumber: 1 tablespoon
- Peeled tomato: ½

OOOOOOOOOOOOOOOOOO

Procedure:

A. Start by blending half of a peeled tomato, 1 tablespoon of crushed cucumber, 2 teaspoons of sour milk, 4 mint leaves, and 3 tablespoons of oatmeal. Blend until you achieve a creamy paste-like consistency.

B. Before applying the peel, ensure that your face and neck are clean and free from any makeup or dirt. You can use a gentle cleanser or face wash to cleanse your skin thoroughly.

C. Using your fingers, apply the prepared paste evenly on your face and neck. Make sure to avoid the delicate area around your eyes.

D. Gently massage the paste onto your skin using circular motions. This helps in promoting blood circulation and ensures even application of the peel.

E. Allow the peel to sit on your skin for a minimum of 10 minutes. During this time, you may experience a cooling and refreshing sensation.

F. After the recommended duration, rinse off the peel using tepid water. Make sure to remove the peel completely from your face and neck.

G. Pat your skin dry with a clean towel and follow up with your regular skincare routine, such as applying moisturizer or sunscreen.

Notes:

A. This tomato and cucumber chemical peel is known for its refreshing and brightening properties, leaving your skin with a healthy glow.

B. If you have any known allergies or sensitivities to the ingredients, it is advisable to perform a patch test on a small area of your skin before applying the peel to your entire face.

C. Adjust the ingredient quantities according to your preference and skin type. For sensitive skin, it is recommended to reduce the amount of oatmeal or mint leaves to avoid any potential irritation.

D. It is recommended to use this peel once or twice a week for best results.

E. Store any leftover paste in an airtight container in the refrigerator for up to 2 days.

4. Grape and Apple Juice

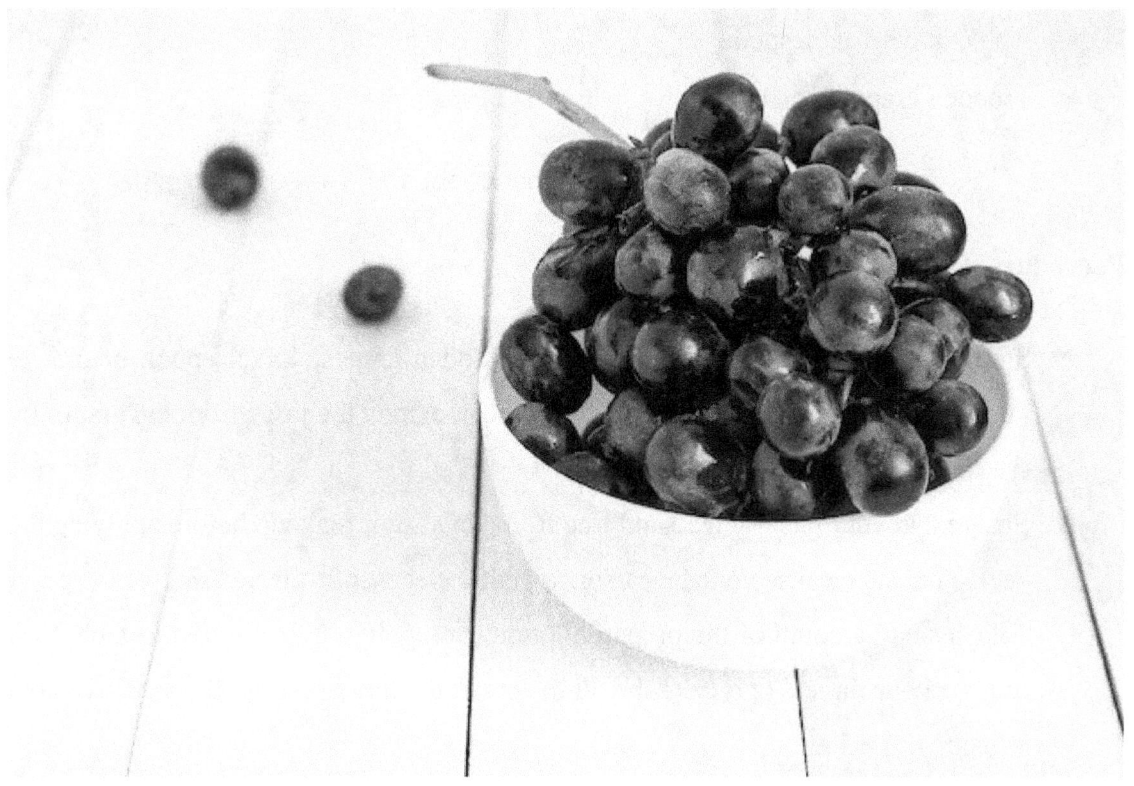

Cooking Time: 5 minutes

Application Time: 10 minutes

List of Ingredients:

- Orange juice: 1 tablespoon
- Apple juice: 1 tablespoon
- Trodden grapes: 6

OOOOOOOOOOOOOOOOOO

Procedure:

A. Start by preparing a natural lotion using trodden grapes, 1 tablespoon of orange juice, and 1 tablespoon of apple juice. You can extract the juice from the grapes by crushing them or using a juicer.

B. Ensure that your face is clean and free from any dirt or makeup before applying the peel. You can cleanse your face using a gentle cleanser or face wash.

C. Take a small amount of the prepared lotion and apply it evenly on your face. You can use your fingers or a clean brush to spread the lotion. Avoid the sensitive area around your eyes.

D. Gently massage the lotion into your skin using circular motions. This helps in promoting blood circulation and ensures that the peel is evenly distributed.

E. Allow the lotion to sit on your face for at least 15 minutes. During this time, you may experience a mild tingling or cooling sensation.

F. After the recommended duration, rinse off the lotion from your face using cold water. Make sure to thoroughly remove all traces of the peel.

G. Pat your skin dry with a clean towel and continue with your regular skincare routine, such as applying moisturizer or sunscreen.

Notes:

A. The grape and apple juice chemical peel is known for its rejuvenating and brightening properties, helping to improve the appearance of your skin.

B. If you have any known allergies to grapes, oranges, or apples, it is advisable to perform a patch test on a small area of your skin before applying the peel to your entire face.

C. Adjust the ingredient quantities according to your preference and skin type. If you have sensitive skin, you may want to dilute the juice with some water to avoid any potential irritation.

D. It is recommended to use this peel once a week for best results.

E. Store any leftover lotion in a sealed container in the refrigerator and use it within a day or two to maintain its freshness and effectiveness.

5. Avocado and Strawberries

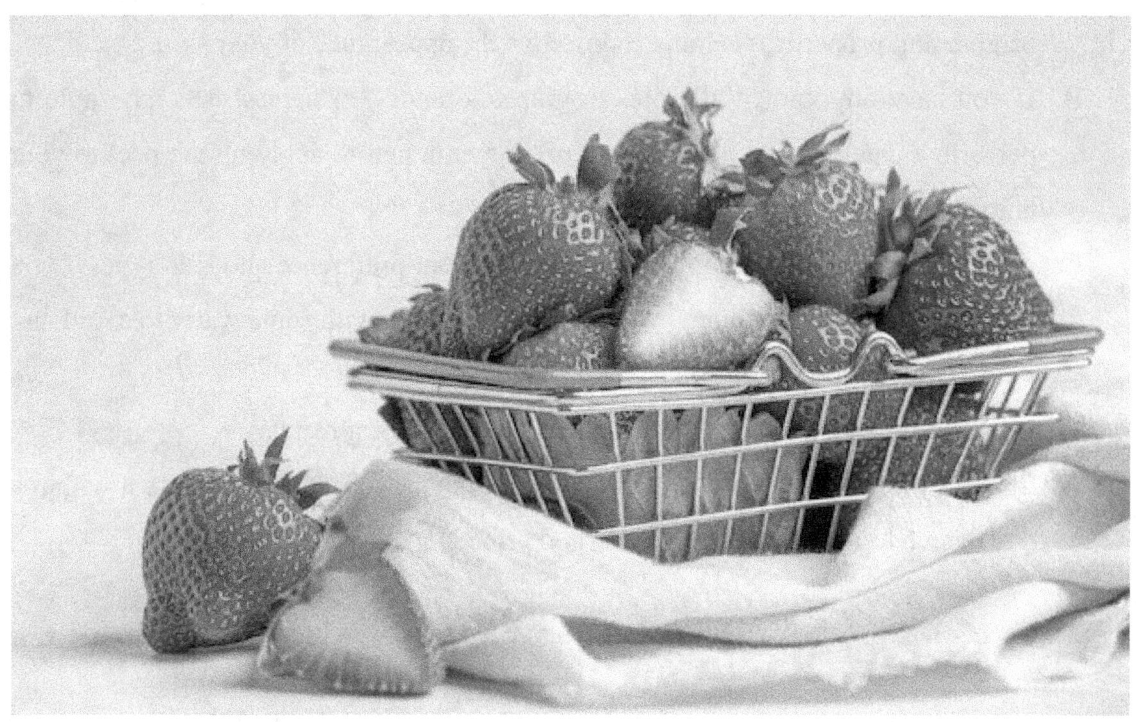

It is a great tonic to take away dead skin layers from your neck and face. This is a tested recipe therefore, you can apply it to your skin without any doubt.

Cooking Time: 5 minutes

Application Time: 20 minutes

List of Ingredients:

- Avocado: 1
- Strawberries: 4

oooooooooooooooooo

Procedure:

A. Start by gathering 1 ripe avocado and 4 fresh strawberries. Ensure that the avocado is properly ripe for easy blending and optimal results.

B. In a blender or food processor, combine the avocado flesh (peeled and pitted) along with the strawberries. Blend the ingredients until you achieve a smooth and creamy consistency. You can also mash the avocado and strawberries together using a fork for a slightly chunkier texture.

C. Before applying the peel, cleanse your face with a gentle cleanser or face wash to remove any impurities and prepare your skin for the treatment.

D. Using clean fingers or a brush, apply a generous layer of the avocado and strawberry mixture to your face, avoiding the eye area. Allow the peel to sit on your skin for approximately 20 minutes. During this time, you can relax and let the nourishing properties of the ingredients work their magic.

E. After the recommended application time, rinse off the peel with cold water. Gently massage your face while rinsing to exfoliate any dead skin cells and enhance the brightening effects.

Notes:

A. The avocado and strawberry chemical peel is a natural and refreshing treatment that can help hydrate and revitalize your skin.

B. Avocado is rich in healthy fats, vitamins, and antioxidants, which can nourish and moisturize the skin, while strawberries contain vitamin C and natural acids that contribute to a brighter complexion.

C. If you have any known allergies to avocados or strawberries, it is advisable to perform a patch test on a small area of your skin before applying the peel to your entire face.

D. Adjust the ingredient quantities based on your desired consistency and coverage. You can add a few drops of water or honey to thin out the mixture if needed.

E. Remember to always use fresh and clean ingredients for the best results.

F. It is recommended to use this peel once or twice a week to maintain healthy and glowing skin.

G. Store any leftover mixture in an airtight container in the refrigerator and use it within a day or two to preserve its freshness and effectiveness.

Natural Remedies to Normalize Oily Skin

Oily skin could be a worrying type of skin because it can alleviate acne. With oily skin, you cannot go to a party as it is very hard to wear makeup on oily skin for long hours. Your oily skin can embarrass you among other people because they pass weird comments on it and as a result, you are left with no choice instead of using harsh chemicals.

Luckily, there are lots of natural and skin-friendly remedies available that can soothe your skin and normalize its oil. These remedies are harmless therefore you can apply these to your skin without any hesitation. Today I am going to share five remedies to normalize your oily skin. These ingredients are easily accessible from your own kitchen:

OOOOOOOOOOOOOOOOOO

6. Cucumber and Lemon Juice

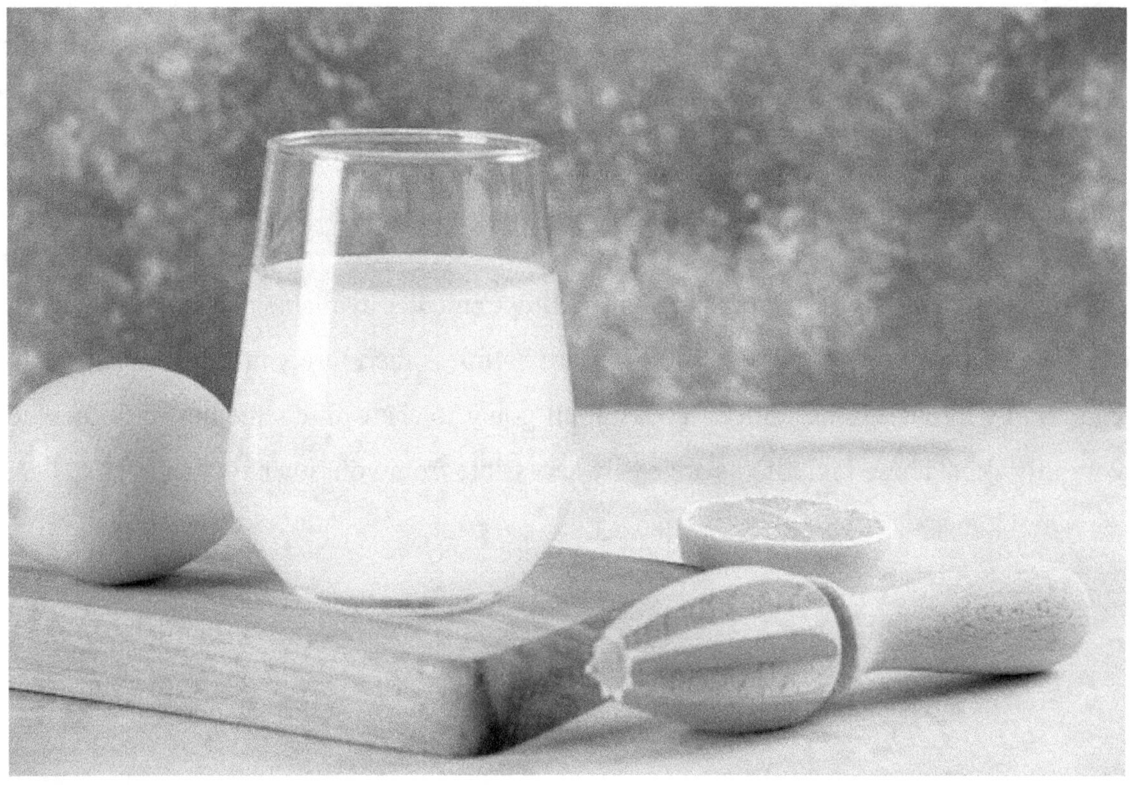

Cucumber and lemon juice are famous to get a fair skin tone and get rid of oily skin. It is very easy to prepare an oily skin healer with the help of these two ingredients.

Cooking Time: 10 minutes

Application Time: 1 hour

List of Ingredients:

- Lemon Juice: 2 tablespoons
- Cucumber: 1 medium

OOOOOOOOOOOOOOOOOO

Procedure:

A. Begin by gathering 1 medium-sized cucumber and 2 tablespoons of lemon juice. These ingredients are excellent for creating a natural remedy to normalize oily skin.

B. Peel and remove the seeds from the cucumber. Using a blender or food processor, blend the cucumber until you obtain a smooth and consistent pulp.

C. In a bowl, combine the cucumber pulp with the 2 tablespoons of lemon juice. Mix the ingredients thoroughly to ensure they are well incorporated. Lemon juice helps to balance the skin's oil production and has astringent properties.

D. Before applying the toner, cleanse your face thoroughly with a gentle cleanser or face wash to remove any dirt or impurities. This step prepares your skin for better absorption of the toner.

E. Dip a cotton ball into the prepared toner mixture and gently apply it to your face, focusing on areas prone to excess oil. Ensure that your entire face is covered with the toner, but avoid getting it into your eyes.

F. Leave the toner on your skin for at least one hour. This allows the natural ingredients to work their magic and regulate the oiliness of your skin. For even better results, you can apply the toner in the evening before going to bed and leave it on overnight.

G. After the recommended application time, rinse off the toner with cool water and pat your skin dry. You will notice a refreshed and less oily complexion.

A. This natural remedy using cucumber and lemon juice is ideal for individuals with oily skin, as it helps to control excess oil and restore balance.

B. Lemon juice acts as a natural astringent, which can tighten pores and reduce oiliness, while cucumber has cooling and soothing properties that can calm and refresh the skin.

C. Make sure to wash your face thoroughly before applying the toner to remove any makeup, dirt, or oils that may hinder its effectiveness.

D. It is recommended to apply the toner in the evening and leave it on overnight for maximum benefits, but if you prefer a shorter application time, one hour is sufficient.

E. Consistency is key for long-term results, so it is advisable to use this toner once everyday or every other day for continuous improvement in oil control.

F. Store any remaining toner in a sealed container in the refrigerator to maintain its freshness. Discard the toner if it develops an unpleasant odor or shows signs of spoilage.

G. If you have sensitive skin or experience any irritation, it is recommended to perform a patch test before applying the toner to your entire face.

H. Remember to protect your skin from excessive sun exposure and use sunscreen daily, as lemon juice can make your skin more sensitive to sunlight.

I. Adjust the ingredient quantities as needed, but maintain the ratio of cucumber pulp to lemon juice for optimal results.

J. Enjoy the benefits of this natural remedy as part of your skincare routine and embrace a healthier, more balanced complexion.

7. Baking Soda and Oatmeal

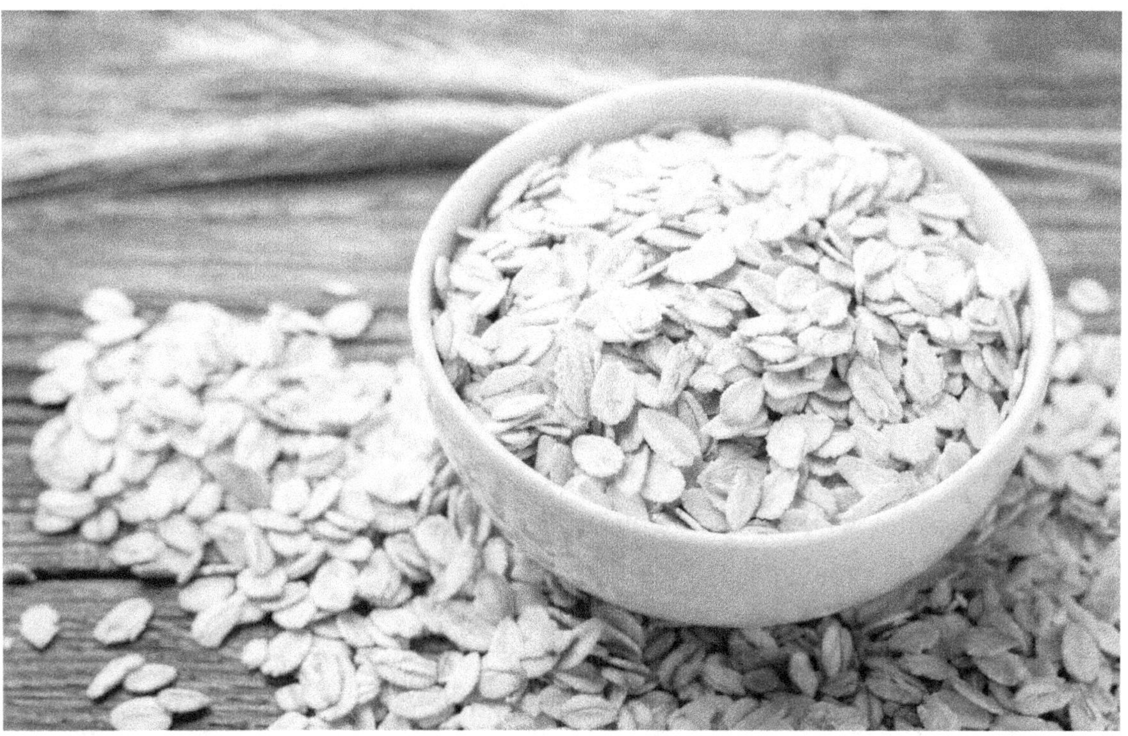

It is the best remedy to get rid of greasy spots on your skin.

Cooking Time: 10 minutes

Application Time: 8 minutes

List of Ingredients:

- Oatmeal: 1 teaspoon
- Water: as per need
- Baking soda: 1 teaspoon

OOOOOOOOOOOOOOOOOO

Procedure:

A. Begin by gathering 1 teaspoon of baking soda and 1 teaspoon of oatmeal. These two ingredients work together to create a natural remedy that helps normalize oily skin.

B. In a small bowl, combine the baking soda and oatmeal. Add a small amount of water gradually while stirring the mixture. The goal is to create a paste with a smooth and spreadable consistency.

C. Before applying the paste, cleanse your face thoroughly using a gentle cleanser or face wash. This step ensures that your skin is free from dirt and impurities, allowing the remedy to work effectively.

D. Using your fingertips, apply the paste to your face, focusing on areas prone to oiliness. Gently massage the paste into your skin in circular motions for 2 to 3 minutes. This helps to exfoliate the skin and unclog pores.

E. Leave the paste on your face for approximately 5 minutes. This allows the ingredients to penetrate the skin and absorb excess oil.

F. After the designated application time, rinse off the paste with cold water. Cold water helps to tighten the pores and refresh the skin.

G. Pat your skin dry with a clean towel. You will notice a reduction in excess oil and a smoother complexion.

Notes:

A. This natural remedy combining baking soda and oatmeal is specifically designed to help normalize oily skin by absorbing excess oil and unclogging pores.

B. Baking soda has natural antiseptic and exfoliating properties, while oatmeal is known for its ability to soothe and nourish the skin.

C. It is important to cleanse your face thoroughly before applying the paste to ensure optimal results.

D. Be gentle when massaging the paste onto your skin, as excessive scrubbing can cause irritation.

E. Adjust the amount of water added to the mixture as needed to achieve the desired paste consistency.

F. Avoid applying the paste to broken or irritated skin, as baking soda may cause further sensitivity.

G. After rinsing off the paste, you may choose to follow up with a gentle moisturizer to keep your skin hydrated.

H. If you experience any discomfort or irritation during or after application, discontinue use and rinse your face with water.

I. Incorporate this natural remedy into your skincare routine as needed to help control excess oil and maintain a balanced complexion.

J. Store any remaining paste in a sealed container for future use, but discard it if it becomes dry or shows signs of spoilage.

K. Remember to patch-test the paste on a small area of your skin before applying it to your entire face, especially if you have sensitive skin.

L. Regular use of this remedy can help improve the appearance of oily skin, but it is important to combine it with a proper skincare routine and a healthy lifestyle for optimal results.

8. Cucumber and Sugar Pack

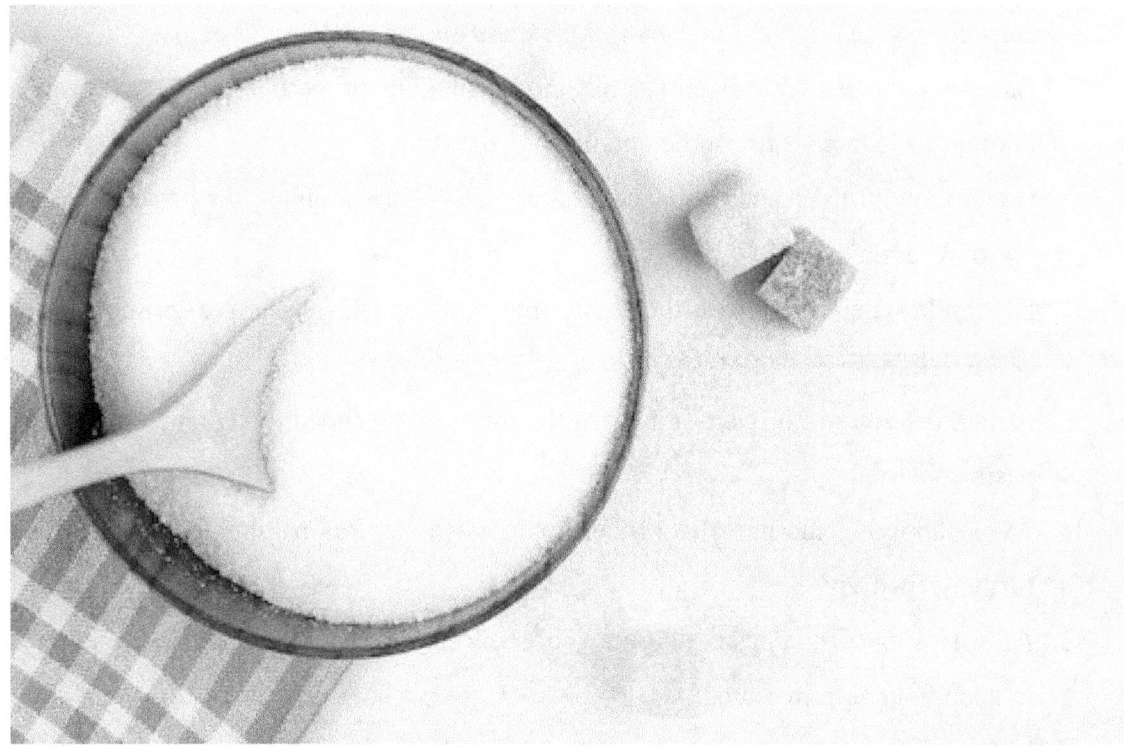

Cucumber is a wonderful and easily accessible ingredient to treat oily skin. It is very easy to prepare cucumber packs for the treatment of oily skin.

Cooking Time: 5 minutes

Application Time: 10 minutes

List of Ingredients:

- Cucumber Juice: crush 1 average cucumber to get its juice
- Sugar: 1 tablespoon

OOOOOOOOOOOOOOOOOO

Procedure:

A. Start by crushing an average-sized cucumber to extract its juice. You can use a blender or a juicer to obtain the cucumber juice.

B. In a small bowl, combine 1 tablespoon of sugar with the cucumber juice. Stir well until the sugar is fully dissolved in the juice. The sugar acts as a natural exfoliant and helps remove dead skin cells.

C. Before applying the pack, cleanse your face thoroughly using a gentle cleanser or face wash. This step ensures that your skin is clean and ready to receive the benefits of the pack.

D. Using clean fingertips or a cotton ball, apply the cucumber and sugar pack to your face. Focus on areas that are prone to oiliness or areas with clogged pores. Gently massage the pack into your skin using circular motions.

E. Allow the pack to sit on your skin for at least 10 minutes. This gives the ingredients time to work and helps absorb excess oil from your skin.

F. After the designated application time, rinse off the pack with cold water. Cold water helps to close the pores and tighten the skin.

G. Pat your skin dry with a clean towel. You will notice a refreshed and mattified complexion.

Notes:

A. This natural remedy combines the soothing properties of cucumber juice with the exfoliating effects of sugar to help normalize oily skin.

B. Cucumber juice is known for its cooling and hydrating properties, making it ideal for oily skin types.

C. Sugar acts as a gentle exfoliant, helping to remove dead skin cells and unclog pores.

D. Make sure to extract enough cucumber juice to achieve a smooth consistency when mixed with sugar. Adjust the amount of sugar as desired, keeping in mind that too much sugar may be harsh on the skin.

E. Cleanse your face before applying the pack to ensure maximum effectiveness.

F. Gently massage the pack into your skin to promote circulation and enhance the exfoliating benefits.

G. Allow the pack to sit on your skin for at least 10 minutes to allow the ingredients to work.

H. Rinse off the pack with cold water to help tighten the pores and give your skin a refreshed feeling.

I. Pat your skin dry instead of rubbing to avoid unnecessary irritation.

J. Use this remedy as needed to help control excess oil and maintain a balanced complexion.

K. If you experience any discomfort or irritation during or after application, discontinue use and rinse your face with water.

L. Incorporate this natural remedy into your skincare routine and complement it with a healthy lifestyle and proper skin care practices for optimal results.

M. Store any leftover cucumber juice and sugar pack in the refrigerator for future use. Discard if it shows signs of spoilage or if the cucumber juice becomes discolored.

N. Conduct a patch test on a small area of your skin before applying the pack to your entire face, especially if you have sensitive skin.

O. Regular use of this remedy, along with a consistent skincare routine, can help improve the appearance of oily skin. However, results may vary depending on individual skin types and conditions.

9. Lemon Juice and Apple Juice Cleanser

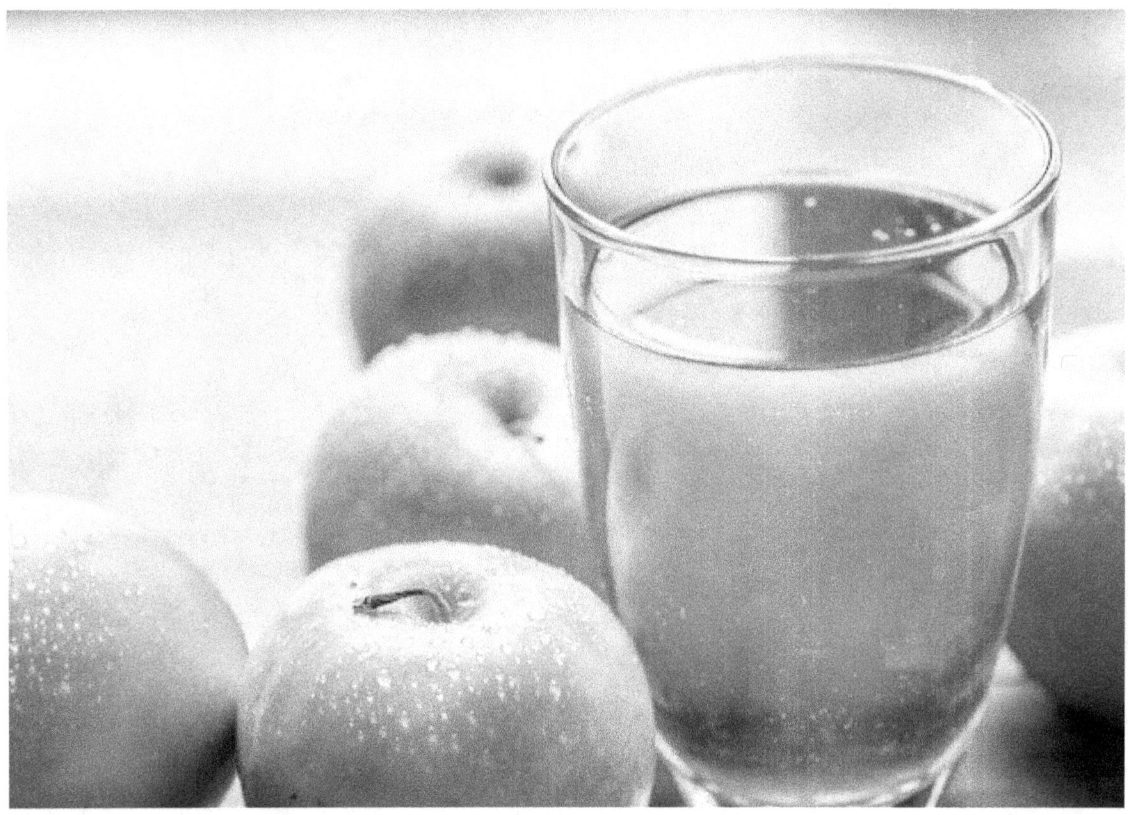

Lemon and apple juice are one of the best cleansers for your skin. It is really easy to get rid of oily skin with 2 tbsp. of lemon juice and two tbsp. of apple juice.

Cooking Time: 5 minutes

Application Time: 15 minutes

List of Ingredients:

- Lemon juice: 2 tablespoons
- Apple Juice: 2 tablespoons

OOOOOOOOOOOOOOOOOO

Procedure:

A. Start by combining 2 tablespoons of lemon juice and 2 tablespoons of apple juice. Lemon juice helps to cleanse and balance the skin, while apple juice contains natural acids that can help control oil production.

B. Before applying the cleanser, ensure your face is clean and free from any makeup or dirt. You can use a gentle cleanser or face wash to cleanse your skin thoroughly.

C. Soak a cotton ball in the lemon and apple juice mixture. Gently apply the cleanser to your face, focusing on areas that are prone to oiliness or areas with clogged pores. You can also apply it to your neck if desired.

D. Allow the cleanser to sit on your skin for at least 15 minutes. This gives the natural acids in the lemon and apple juice time to work and helps normalize oily skin.

E. After the designated application time, rinse off the cleanser with cold water. The cold water helps to tighten the pores and leaves your skin feeling refreshed.

F. Pat your skin dry with a clean towel. Avoid rubbing your face to prevent unnecessary irritation.

G. For optimal results, use this natural cleanser at least once a day. Consistency is key, so continue using it for a few weeks to see improvements in your skin's oiliness.

Notes:

A. This natural remedy combines the cleansing properties of lemon juice with the natural acids found in apple juice to help normalize oily skin.

B. Lemon juice is known for its astringent properties, which can help control oil production and reduce the appearance of enlarged pores.

C. Apple juice contains natural fruit acids, such as malic acid, which can exfoliate the skin and improve its texture.

D. Before applying the cleanser, make sure your face is clean and free from any makeup or dirt. This ensures maximum effectiveness.

E. Soak a cotton ball in the lemon and apple juice mixture and gently apply it to your face. You can also use a cotton pad or your fingertips if preferred.

F. Allow the cleanser to sit on your skin for at least 15 minutes to allow the natural acids to work.

G. Rinse off the cleanser with cold water to help tighten the pores and give your skin a refreshed feeling.

H. Pat your skin dry instead of rubbing to avoid unnecessary irritation.

I. Use this cleanser at least once a day as part of your skincare routine to help control excess oil and maintain a balanced complexion.

J. Consistency is important, so continue using the cleanser for a few weeks to see improvements in your skin's oiliness.

K. If you experience any discomfort or irritation during or after application, discontinue use and rinse your face with water.

L. Conduct a patch test on a small area of your skin before applying the cleanser to your entire face, especially if you have sensitive skin.

M. Results may vary depending on individual skin types and conditions. It's important to listen to your skin and adjust the frequency of use as needed.

N. Remember to complement this natural remedy with a healthy lifestyle, proper skin care practices, and a balanced diet for optimal results.

O. Store any leftover lemon and apple juice mixture in a sealed container in the refrigerator for future use. Discard if it shows signs of spoilage.

P. As with any new skincare product, it's recommended to consult with a dermatologist or skin care professional if you have any concerns or specific skin conditions.

10. Oatmeal and Cucumber Face Pack

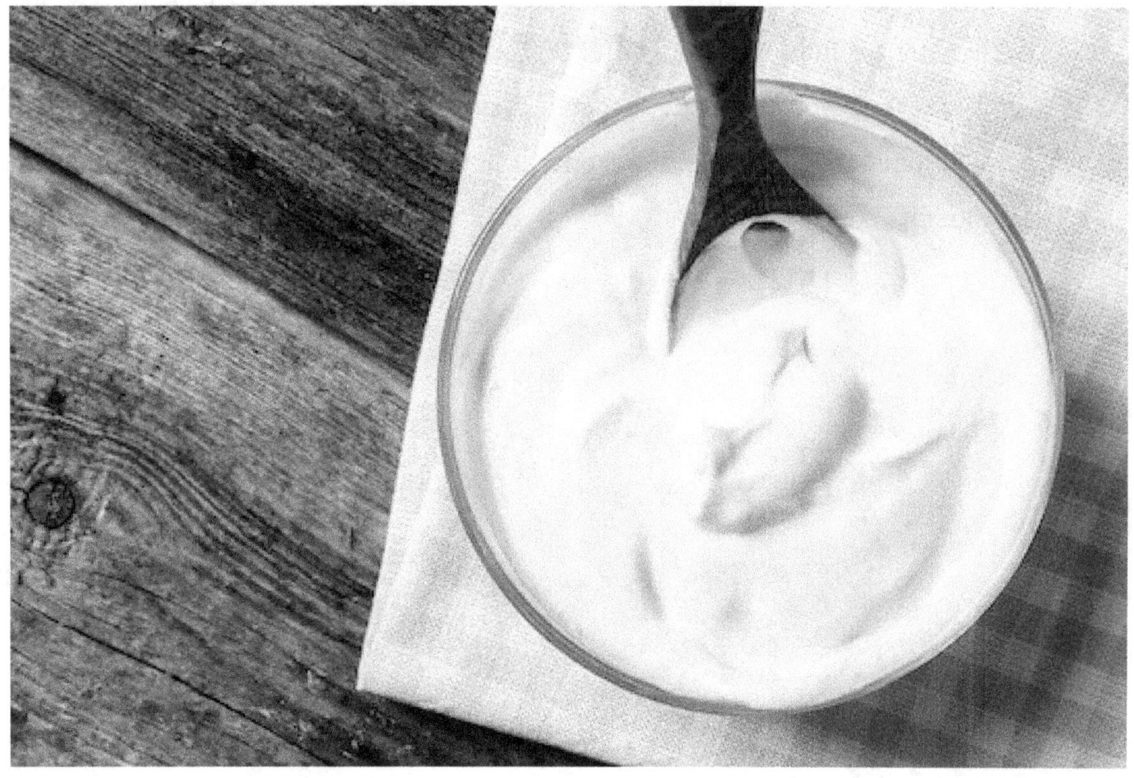

Oatmeal and cucumber can help you in a better way to prevent oil and acne.

Cooking Time: 5 minutes

Application Time: 30 minutes

List of Ingredients:

- Oatmeal: 1 cup
- Yogurt: 2 tablespoons
- Cucumber: 1 small

ooooooooooooooooooo

Procedure:

A. Start by preparing the ingredients. Take 1 cup of oatmeal and 1 small-sized cucumber. Using a blender, blend the cucumber until it forms a smooth puree. Set aside.

B. In a mixing bowl, combine the oatmeal and cucumber puree. Add 2 tablespoons of yogurt to the mixture. Yogurt helps to soothe and nourish the skin.

C. Mix the ingredients well until they form a thick paste. If the consistency is too thick, you can add a small amount of water to achieve the desired texture. The oatmeal will provide gentle exfoliation while the cucumber helps to balance the skin.

D. Before applying the face pack, ensure your face is clean and free from any makeup or dirt. You can use a gentle cleanser or face wash to cleanse your skin thoroughly.

E. Using clean fingers or a face mask brush, apply the oatmeal and cucumber face pack evenly on your face, avoiding the delicate eye area. You can also apply it on your neck if desired.

F. Leave the face pack on for approximately 30 minutes. During this time, the oatmeal will help absorb excess oil and impurities, while the cucumber provides a cooling and refreshing effect.

G. After the designated application time, rinse off the face pack with lukewarm water. Gently massage the pack into your skin as you rinse to maximize its exfoliating benefits. Pat your skin dry with a clean towel.

Notes:

A. This natural face pack combines the exfoliating properties of oatmeal with the soothing and balancing effects of cucumber and yogurt.

B. Oatmeal acts as a gentle exfoliant, helping to remove dead skin cells and unclog pores, resulting in a smoother complexion.

C. Cucumber is known for its cooling and hydrating properties, which can help soothe and reduce inflammation in the skin.

D. Yogurt contains lactic acid, which helps to exfoliate and brighten the skin, while also providing moisture and nourishment.

E. Before applying the face pack, ensure your face is clean and free from any makeup or dirt. This allows the ingredients to penetrate and work effectively.

F. Mix the oatmeal, cucumber puree, and yogurt thoroughly to form a thick paste. Adjust the consistency by adding a small amount of water if needed.

G. Apply the face pack evenly to your face, avoiding the delicate eye area. You can also extend it to your neck for a complete treatment.

H. Leave the face pack on for approximately 30 minutes to allow the ingredients to work their magic. Relax and enjoy the cooling sensation.

I. After the designated application time, rinse off the face pack with lukewarm water. Gently massage the pack into your skin as you rinse to maximize its exfoliating benefits.

J. Pat your skin dry with a clean towel instead of rubbing to avoid unnecessary irritation.

K. For best results, use this face pack regularly as part of your skincare routine. Consistency is key to achieving and maintaining balanced and healthy-looking skin.

L. Remember to listen to your skin and adjust the frequency of use if needed. If you experience any discomfort or irritation, discontinue use and rinse your face with water.

M. As with any new skincare product, it's recommended to conduct a patch test on a small area of your skin before applying the face pack to your entire face, especially if you have sensitive skin.

N. Results may vary depending on individual skin types and conditions. It's important to observe how your skin responds to the ingredients and adjust accordingly.

O. Store any leftover face pack in a sealed container in the refrigerator for future use. Discard if it shows signs of spoilage.

P. Complement this natural remedy with a healthy lifestyle, proper skin care practices, and a balanced diet for optimal results.

Q. If you have any concerns or specific skin conditions, it's advisable to consult with a dermatologist or skincare professional.

Tested Home Remedies for Blackheads

Sebaceous glands are awfully vigorous glands and responsible for oily skin. Excess oil can block the pores of your skin which leads to lots of skin problems. Blackheads are one of the famous skin problems and in the presence of blackheads, your skin requires deep cleansing treatment on a regular basis. Tiny black spots on the nose, cheek, and forehead look very ugly and can spoil your whole style. It is really necessary to treat these tiny black spots as early as possible otherwise this problem could get worse in the near future. No need to rush to medical stores or dermatologists because some grocery items are enough for the best treatment. Today I will share some easy recipes to treat your blackheads:

OOOOOOOOOOOOOOOOOO

11. Almond Powder and Rose Water

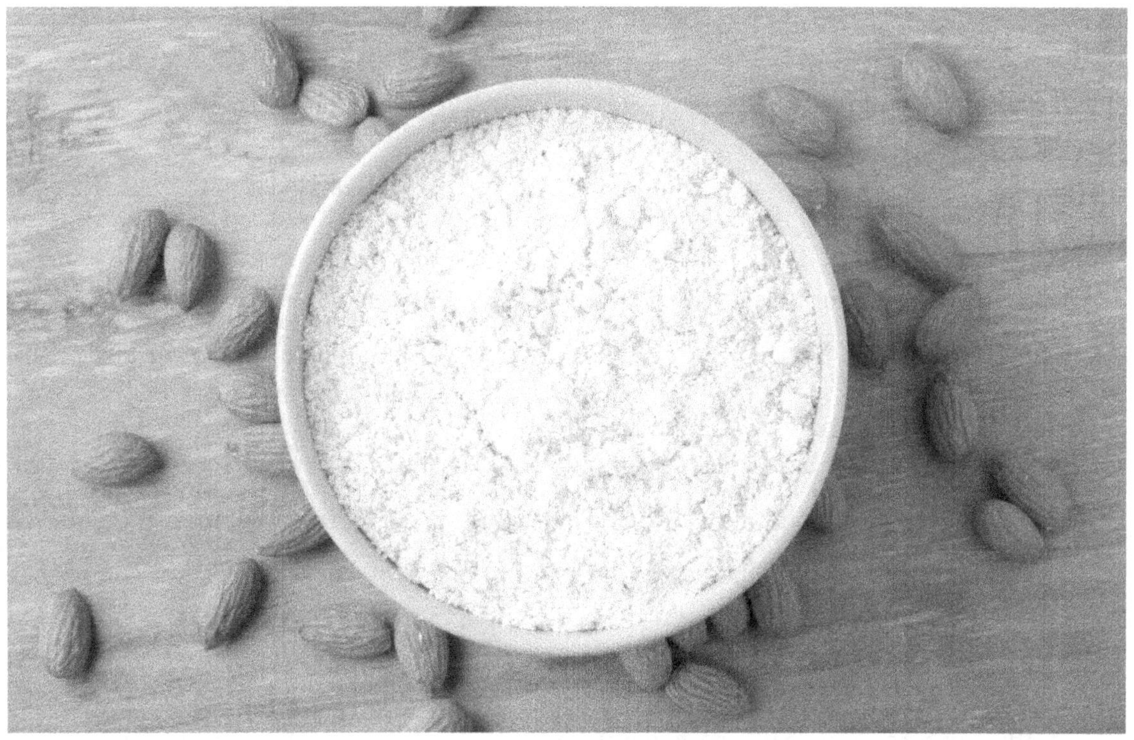

Almond powder and rose water are the best to get deep cleansing facial treatment for your skin toning.

Cooking Time: 5 minutes

Application Time: 15 minutes

List of Ingredients:

- Rose water: as needed
- Almond powder: 5 teaspoons

OOOOOOOOOOOOOOOOOO

Procedure:

A. Start by gathering the ingredients needed for this home remedy: almond powder and rose water. You will need approximately 5 teaspoons of almond powder and enough rose water to create a paste-like consistency.

B. In a small bowl, combine the almond powder and rose water. Gradually add the rose water to the almond powder while stirring continuously until you achieve a smooth paste. Adjust the amount of rose water as needed to create a spreadable consistency.

C. Ensure your face is clean and free from any makeup or impurities before applying the mixture. You can use a gentle cleanser or face wash to cleanse your skin thoroughly. Pat dry with a clean towel.

D. Using your fingertips, apply the almond powder and rose water mixture to your face, focusing on areas prone to blackheads. Gently massage the mixture into your skin using circular motions. The almond powder acts as a natural exfoliant, helping to remove dead skin cells and unclog pores.

E. Allow the mask to sit on your skin for approximately 15 minutes. During this time, the mixture will work to draw out impurities and tighten the pores. Take this opportunity to relax and enjoy the soothing properties of rose water.

F. After the designated application time, rinse off the mask with cold water. The cold water helps to tighten the pores and provides a refreshing finish. Gently pat your skin dry with a clean towel.

G. For optimal results, repeat this remedy three times a week. Consistency is key to effectively targeting blackheads and promoting clearer skin. Over time, you should notice a visible improvement in the appearance of blackheads.

Notes:

A. This homemade remedy utilizes the exfoliating properties of almond powder and the soothing benefits of rose water to address blackheads.

B. The almond powder acts as a gentle exfoliator, helping to remove dead skin cells and unclog pores. It also contains natural oils that nourish and moisturize the skin.

C. Rose water has anti-inflammatory properties and helps to soothe irritated skin. It also aids in balancing the skin's pH levels and tightening the pores.

D. Before applying the mixture, ensure your face is clean and free from any makeup or impurities. This allows the ingredients to penetrate the skin more effectively.

E. Gradually add the rose water to the almond powder while stirring to achieve the desired consistency. The mixture should form a smooth paste that is easy to spread on the skin.

F. Apply the mixture to your face, focusing on areas where blackheads are commonly found, such as the nose, chin, and forehead.

G. Gently massage the mixture into your skin using circular motions. This helps to exfoliate the skin and enhance the removal of dead skin cells and impurities.

H. Allow the mask to sit on your skin for approximately 15 minutes. This allows the ingredients to work their magic and draw out impurities from the pores.

I. Rinse off the mask with cold water. The cold water helps to tighten the pores and provides a refreshing sensation to the skin.

J. Pat your skin dry with a clean towel instead of rubbing it to avoid unnecessary irritation.

K. For optimal results, repeat this remedy three times a week. Consistency is key to effectively targeting blackheads and maintaining clearer skin.

L. It's important to note that results may vary depending on individual skin types and conditions. It's recommended to observe how your skin responds to the ingredients and adjust accordingly.

M. If you have sensitive skin or any existing skin conditions, it's advisable to perform a patch test before applying the mixture to your entire face.

N. Store any leftover almond powder and rose water mixture in a sealed container for future use. Discard if it shows signs of spoilage.

O. Complement this home remedy with a healthy skincare routine, including regular cleansing and moisturizing, as well as a balanced diet and proper hydration for overall skin health.

12. Pomegranate Skin and Lime Juice

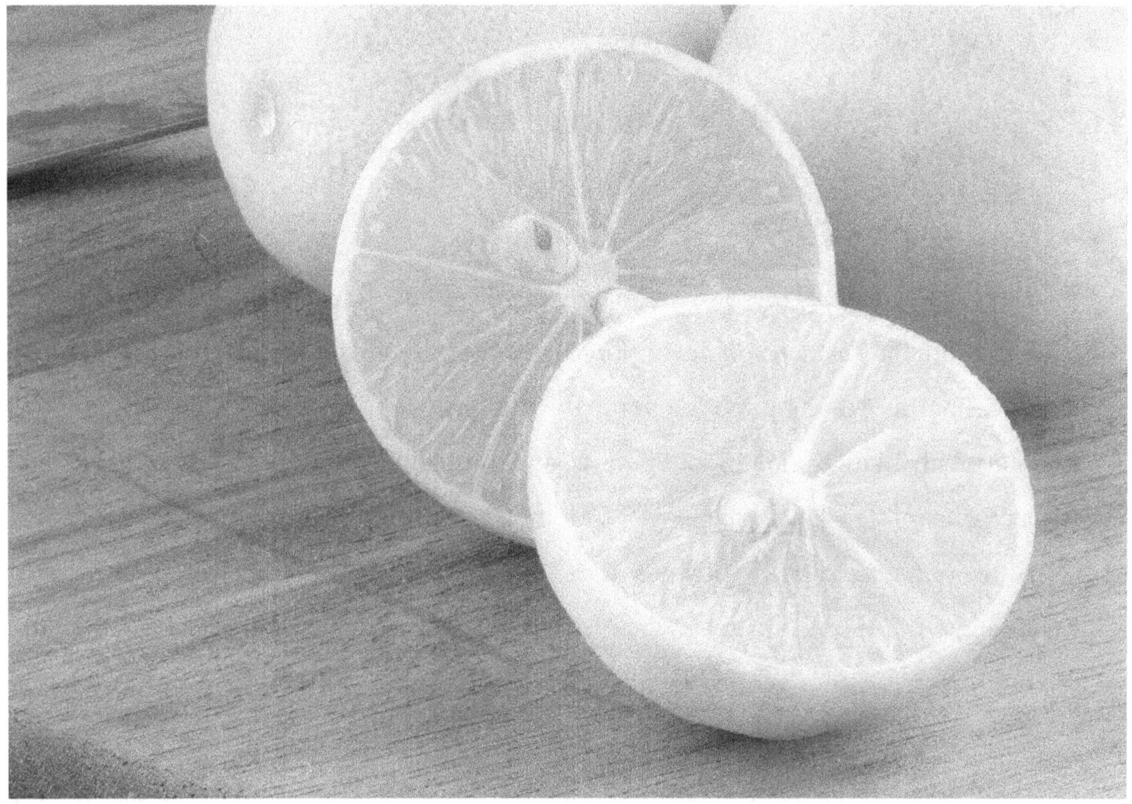

Pomegranate is highly recommended to those who want to treat their skin complexion.

Cooking Time: 5 minutes

Application Time: 10 minutes

List of Ingredients:

- Pomegranate skin powder: 2 tablespoons
- Lemon Juice: 1 tablespoon or more

OOOOOOOOOOOOOOOOOO

Procedure:

A. Begin by crushing the pomegranate skin to obtain fine particles. You will need approximately 2 tablespoons of pomegranate skin powder for this remedy.

B. In a small bowl, combine the pomegranate skin powder with natural lemon juice. Start with 1 tablespoon of lemon juice and gradually add more if needed to achieve a creamy paste-like consistency. The lemon juice helps to enhance the effectiveness of the pomegranate skin powder in treating blackheads.

C. Ensure your face is clean and free from any makeup or impurities before applying the mixture. Use a gentle cleanser or face wash to cleanse your skin thoroughly, and pat it dry with a clean towel.

D. Using clean fingers or a small spatula, apply the pomegranate skin and lemon juice mixture directly onto the areas affected by blackheads. Focus on these areas and gently massage the mixture into the skin. The abrasive texture of the pomegranate skin powder helps to exfoliate the skin and unclog pores, while the lemon juice provides astringent properties.

E. Allow the mixture to sit on your skin for approximately 10 minutes. During this time, the combination of pomegranate skin powder and lemon juice will work to dissolve and remove blackheads. You may feel a slight tingling sensation, which is normal.

F. After the designated application time, dampen a soft cloth with water. Gently wipe away the paste from your skin using the cloth. Be gentle to avoid causing any irritation or redness.

G. To maximize the benefits of this home remedy, rinse your face with cold water to tighten the pores. Pat your skin dry with a clean towel, and follow up with your regular skincare routine.

Notes:

A. Pomegranate skin powder, known for its antioxidant properties, is effective in treating blackheads and promoting healthier skin.

B. Crush the pomegranate skin thoroughly to obtain fine particles. You can use a mortar and pestle or a food processor to achieve a powdered consistency.

C. Combine the pomegranate skin powder with natural lemon juice, which acts as an astringent and helps to remove excess oil and dirt from the pores.

D. Start with 1 tablespoon of lemon juice and adjust the amount as needed to create a creamy paste-like consistency. The paste should be easy to spread on the skin.

E. Ensure your face is clean and dry before applying the mixture. This allows the ingredients to penetrate the skin effectively.

F. Gently massage the paste onto the areas affected by blackheads, using circular motions. This helps to exfoliate the skin and remove impurities from the pores.

G. Allow the mixture to sit on your skin for approximately 10 minutes. This gives the pomegranate skin powder and lemon juice enough time to work on dissolving and removing blackheads.

H. After the designated application time, use a damp, soft cloth to gently wipe away the paste from your skin. Be gentle to avoid any irritation or redness.

I. Rinse your face with cold water to tighten the pores and remove any residue. This step provides a refreshing finish and helps to minimize the appearance of pores.

J. Pat your skin dry with a clean towel. Avoid rubbing, as it can cause irritation.

K. Incorporate this remedy into your skincare routine up to three times a week for optimal results. Consistency is key in treating and preventing blackheads.

L. It's important to note that individual skin types and conditions may vary. If you have sensitive skin or any existing skin conditions, it's advisable to perform a patch test before applying the mixture to your entire face.

M. Store any remaining pomegranate skin powder in a sealed container for future use. Ensure it is kept in a cool, dry place away from direct sunlight.

13. Coriander Leaves and Turmeric Powder Scrub

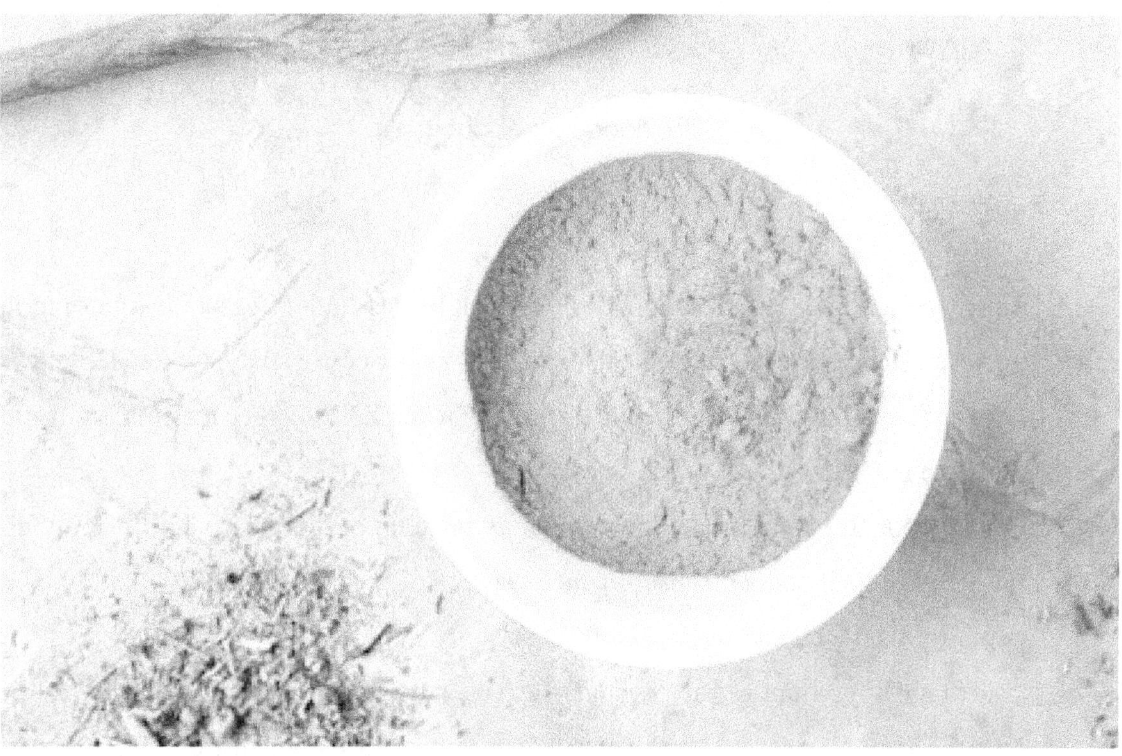

The scrub is the best remedy to eradicate blackheads from your skin. It is very easy to prepare a fine paste with the help of both ingredients.

Cooking Time: 5 minutes

Application Time: 10 minutes

List of Ingredients:

- Turmeric powder: 1 teaspoon
- Coriander leaves: 1 tablespoon

OOOOOOOOOOOOOOOOOO

Procedure:

A. Start by blending 1 tablespoon of coriander leaves and 1 teaspoon of turmeric powder. Blend until you achieve a smooth paste-like consistency. Coriander leaves have antibacterial properties, while turmeric powder helps reduce inflammation and unclog pores.

B. Ensure your face is clean and free from any makeup or impurities before applying the scrub. Use a gentle cleanser or face wash to cleanse your skin thoroughly, and pat it dry with a clean towel.

C. Take a small amount of the coriander leaves and turmeric paste and gently rub it onto the areas affected by blackheads. Focus on these areas and use circular motions to massage the scrub into the skin. The gentle exfoliation from the coriander leaves will help remove dead skin cells and unclog pores, while the turmeric powder will provide anti-inflammatory properties.

D. Allow the scrub to sit on your skin for 5 to 6 minutes. During this time, the mixture will work to cleanse and purify your skin, targeting blackheads and other impurities.

E. After the designated application time, use cold water to thoroughly rinse off the scrub from your face. The cool temperature of the water will help tighten the pores and provide a refreshing finish.

F. Pat your skin dry with a clean towel. Avoid rubbing, as it can cause irritation.

G. For optimal results, use this scrub once a day as part of your skincare routine. Consistency is key in treating and preventing blackheads. Over time, you should notice a reduction in blackheads and a healthier complexion.

Notes:

A. Blend the coriander leaves and turmeric powder together until you achieve a smooth paste. You can add a small amount of water if needed to help with the blending process.

B. Ensure your face is clean and dry before applying the scrub. This allows the ingredients to penetrate the skin effectively.

C. Gently massage the scrub onto the areas affected by blackheads, using circular motions. Focus on areas prone to blackheads, such as the nose, chin, and forehead.

D. Allow the scrub to sit on your skin for 5 to 6 minutes. This allows the ingredients to work on cleansing the pores and removing blackheads.

E. Rinse off the scrub thoroughly with cold water. The cool temperature helps to close the pores and provides a refreshing sensation.

F. Pat your skin dry with a clean towel. Avoid rubbing, as it can cause irritation.

G. Incorporate this scrub into your daily skincare routine for the best results. Consistency is key in treating and preventing blackheads.

H. It's important to note that individual skin types and conditions may vary. If you have sensitive skin or any existing skin conditions, it's advisable to perform a patch test before applying the scrub to your entire face.

I. Store any leftover coriander leaves and turmeric powder scrub in a sealed container in the refrigerator. It is recommended to use the scrub within a few days to maintain its freshness and effectiveness.

14. Witch Hazel Cleanser

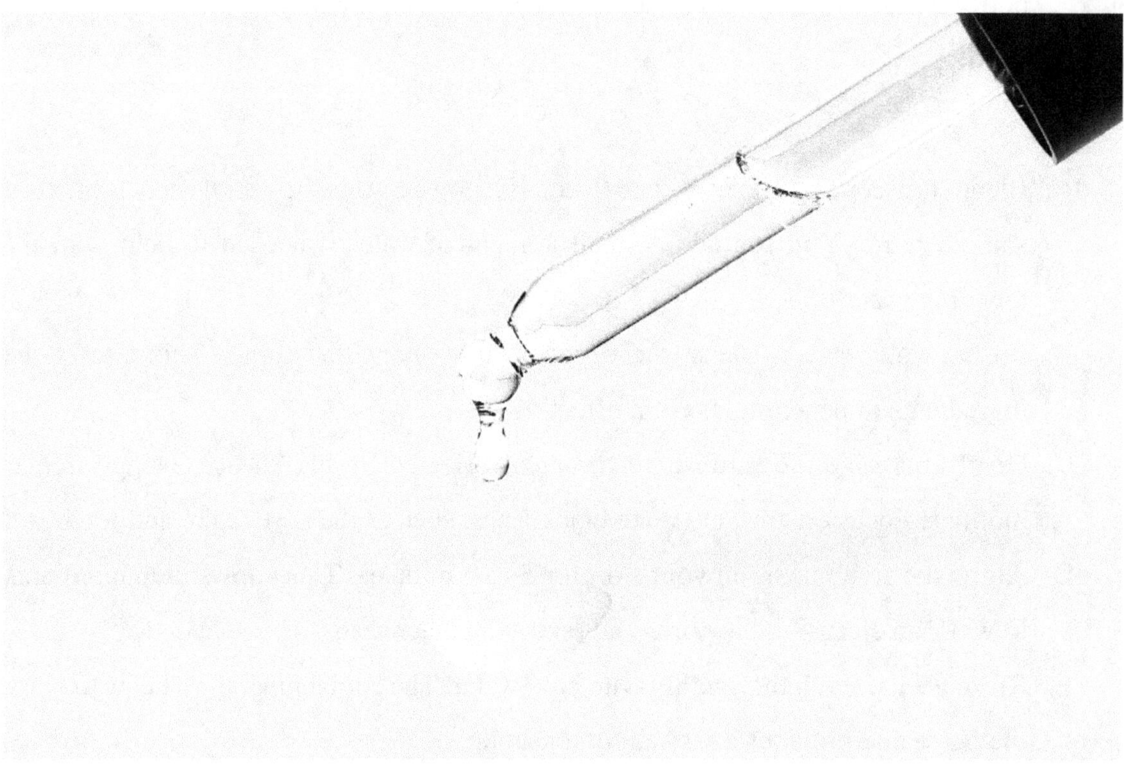

If you want to increase the resistance of your skin against different skin problems then it is good to cleanse it with a few drops of witch hazel.

Cooking Time: 5 minutes

Application Time: 10 minutes

List of Ingredients:

- Witch Hazel: A few drops

OOOOOOOOOOOOOOOOOO

Procedure:

A. Take a cotton pad and apply a few drops of witch hazel onto it. Witch hazel is a natural astringent that helps to cleanse the skin and remove excess oil, dirt, and impurities from the pores.
B. Gently wipe the cotton pad across your face, focusing on areas prone to blackheads or areas where you have clogged pores. This will help to remove any buildup and unclog the pores, preventing the formation of blackheads.
C. Allow the witch hazel to dry on your skin for a few minutes. There is no need to rinse it off, as it will continue to work on your skin and provide a refreshed and clarified appearance.

A. Witch hazel is a natural ingredient known for its astringent properties. It helps to tighten the skin and minimize the appearance of pores.

B. When using witch hazel, ensure that you are using a pure and alcohol-free formulation to avoid any potential skin irritation.

C. Witch hazel can be used as a daily cleanser to maintain clear and blackhead-free skin. However, if you have sensitive skin, it's advisable to start with a patch test before applying it to your entire face.

D. Witch hazel can also be used as a toner after cleansing your face. Simply apply it with a cotton pad and swipe it across your face to remove any remaining impurities and balance the skin's pH levels.

E. For best results, incorporate witch hazel into your daily skincare routine. Consistency is key in preventing and treating blackheads.

F. It's important to note that individual skin types and conditions may vary. If you experience any irritation or discomfort while using witch hazel, discontinue use and consult a dermatologist.

G. Store witch hazel in a cool, dry place away from direct sunlight to maintain its potency and effectiveness.

H. Witch hazel can also be combined with other natural ingredients, such as tea tree oil or apple cider vinegar, for enhanced cleansing and clarifying benefits. However, it's essential to do a patch test and research any potential side effects before combining ingredients.

I. Remember to follow a comprehensive skincare routine that includes cleansing, exfoliating, and moisturizing to maintain healthy, blackhead-free skin.

15. Salty Water Cleanser

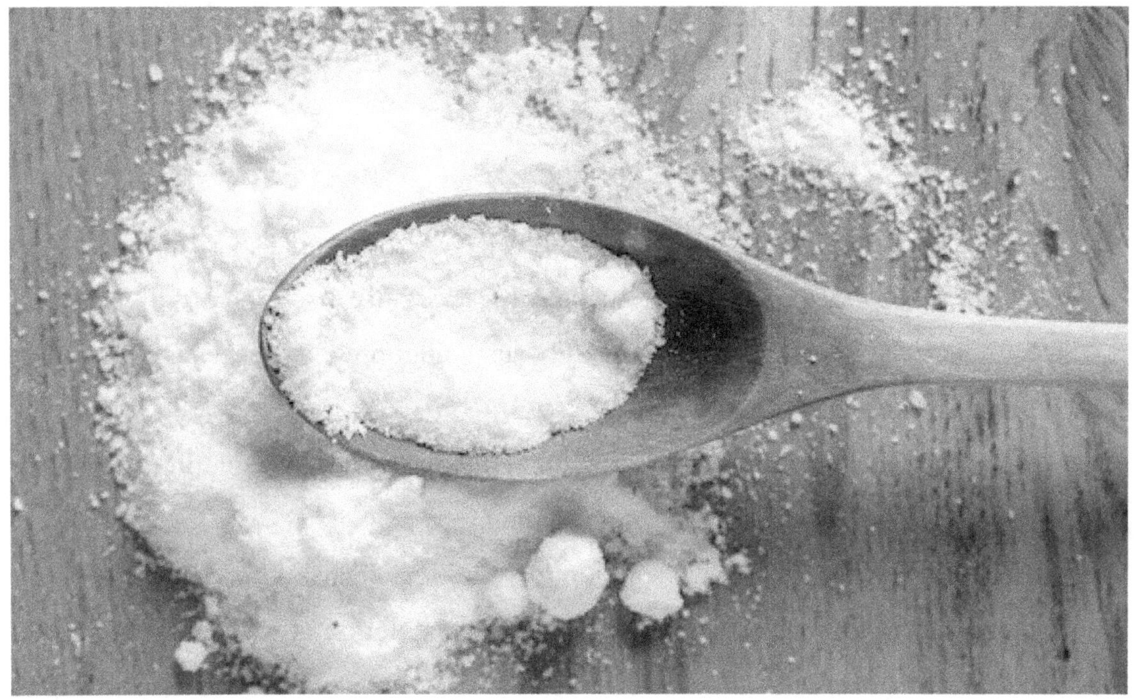

Use of salty water is the best way to cleanse your pores and kick off blackheads. It is very easy to prepare.

Cooking Time: 5 minutes

Application Time: 10 minutes

List of Ingredients:

- Water: 2 tablespoons
- Salt: 1 teaspoon

OOOOOOOOOOOOOOOOOO

Procedure:

A. In a small bowl, combine 2 tablespoons of water with 1 teaspoon of salt. Mix well until the salt is fully dissolved. The saltwater solution will act as a natural cleanser to help cleanse and unclog your skin pores.

B. Take a cotton swab or cotton pad and dip it into the salty water solution. Make sure the cotton swab is saturated but not dripping.

C. Gently apply the salty water solution to your skin, focusing on areas where you have blackheads or clogged pores. Massage the solution into your skin in gentle, circular motions. The salt will help to exfoliate the skin and remove any buildup of dirt, oil, and dead skin cells.

D. Leave the salty water solution on your skin for about 5-10 minutes to allow it to work its cleansing magic. After the designated time, rinse your face with lukewarm water to remove the solution.

A. Saltwater has natural antibacterial properties and can help to cleanse the skin and remove impurities. It also acts as a gentle exfoliant, helping to slough off dead skin cells and unclog pores.

B. When preparing the salty water solution, it's important to use clean, filtered water and pure, non-iodized salt. Iodized salt may cause irritation to the skin.

C. While using the salty water cleanser, it's important to avoid contact with the eyes, as saltwater can be irritating to the delicate eye area.

D. Incorporate this cleansing method into your daily skincare routine for the best results. However, if you have sensitive skin, it's advisable to start with a patch test before applying the solution to your entire face.

E. After cleansing with the salty water solution, it's recommended to follow up with a moisturizer to hydrate and nourish your skin.

F. If you experience any irritation or discomfort while using the salty water solution, discontinue use and consult a dermatologist.

Organic Facials for Normal Skin

OOOOOOOOOOOOOOOOOO

16. Vegetables for suppleness of your skin

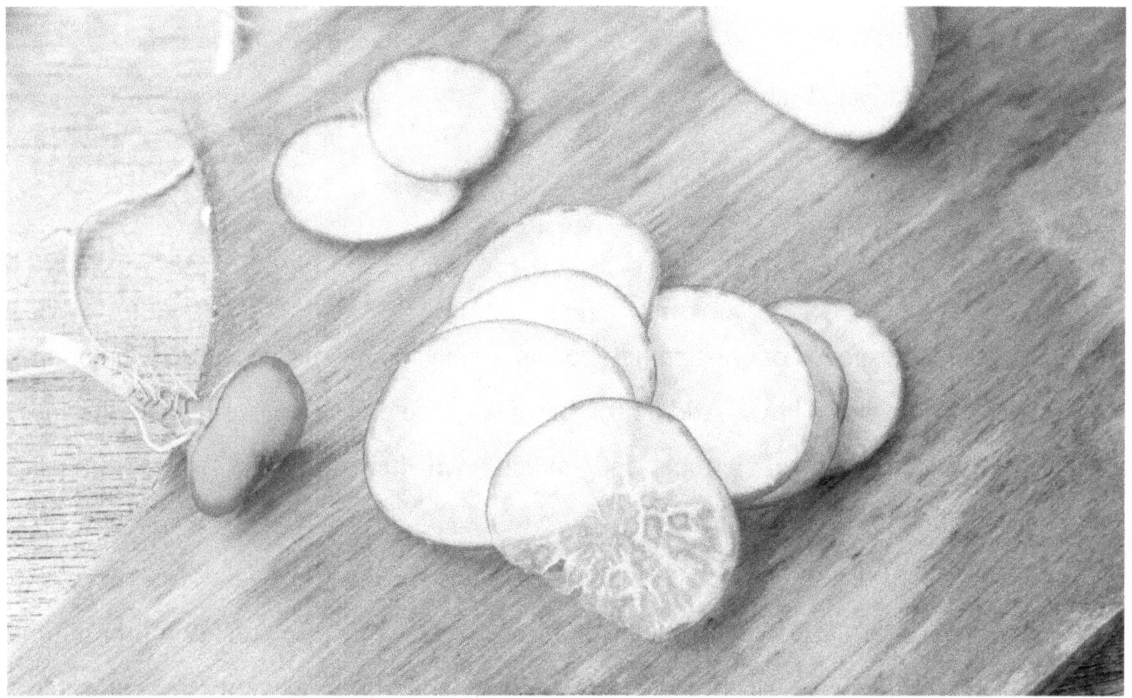

Apply these vegetables to your skin for lots of benefits.

Cooking Time: 5 minutes

Application Time: 15 minutes

List of Ingredients:

- Crushed lettuce: 3 tablespoons
- Water: a little bit
- Crushed Radish: 3 tablespoons

ooooooooooooooooo

Procedure:

A. Take 3 tablespoons of crushed lettuce and 3 tablespoons of crushed radish and mix them together in a bowl. Add a little bit of water to create a paste-like consistency. The combination of lettuce and radish will help promote suppleness and nourishment for your skin.

B. Before applying the mixture, make sure your face is clean and free from any makeup or dirt. Use a gentle cleanser or face wash to cleanse your skin thoroughly.

C. Using clean fingers or a brush, apply the vegetable mixture evenly onto your face, focusing on areas where you have blackheads or areas that need extra nourishment. Gently massage the mixture into your skin in circular motions to promote absorption.

D. Leave the mixture on your face for approximately 15 minutes to allow the nutrients from the vegetables to penetrate your skin and provide their beneficial effects.

E. After the designated time, rinse your face with lukewarm water. Ensure that all the mixture is thoroughly washed off and there is no residue left on your skin.

F. It is recommended to use this vegetable mixture once a week as part of your skincare routine. Consistent usage will help promote a healthy complexion and improve the suppleness of your skin.

Notes:

A. Crushed lettuce and radish are rich in vitamins, minerals, and antioxidants, which can help nourish and rejuvenate the skin.

B. Ensure that the vegetables are thoroughly crushed to create a smooth paste. You can use a blender or food processor to achieve the desired consistency.

C. When mixing the vegetables with water, add just enough water to create a paste. The consistency should be thick enough to adhere to your face without dripping.

D. Before applying the mixture, it is advisable to perform a patch test on a small area of your skin to check for any potential allergies or irritations.

E. While the mixture is on your face, you can relax and indulge in a soothing experience. Consider playing calming music or engaging in a brief meditation to enhance the relaxation and rejuvenation process.

F. If you have any specific skin concerns or conditions, it is recommended to consult a dermatologist before trying any homemade remedies.

G. Remember, everyone's skin is unique, and results may vary. Listen to your skin and adjust the frequency and ingredients of your skincare routine accordingly.

H. Along with using this vegetable mixture, maintaining a balanced diet, staying hydrated, and practicing good skincare habits will contribute to overall skin health.

I. If you experience any adverse reactions or discomfort while using this mixture, discontinue use and seek medical advice.

17. Mango and Papaya

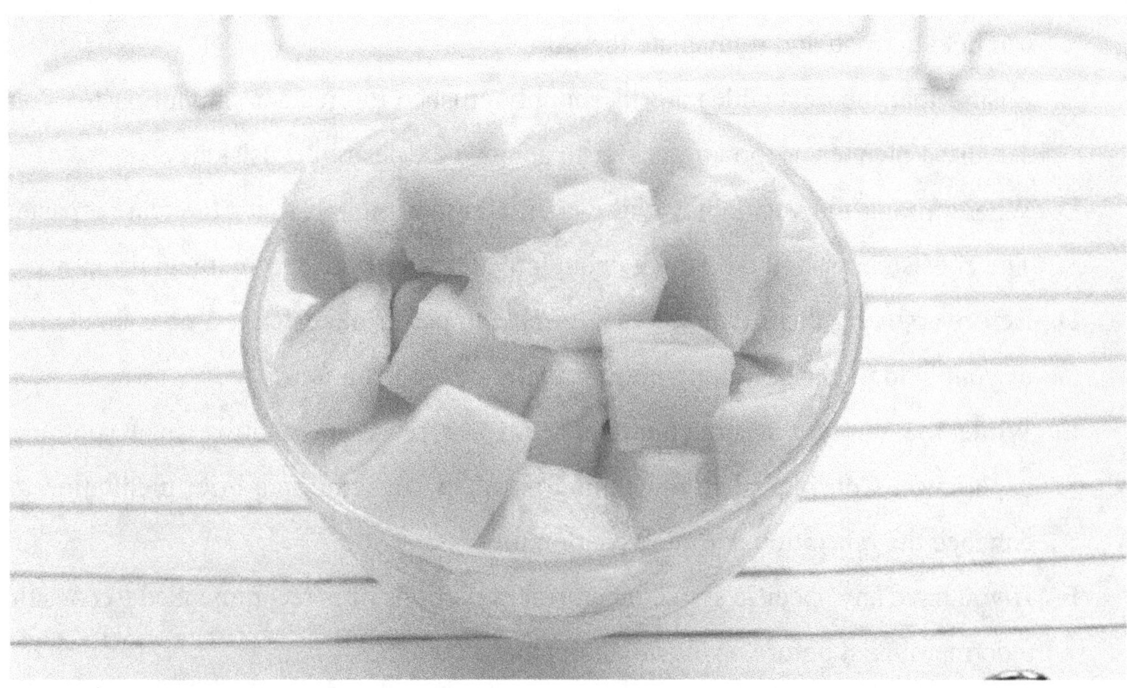

Use mango and papaya to moisturize your skin. This remedy will be a good choice for normal skin.

Cooking Time: 5 minutes

Application Time: 10 minutes

List of Ingredients:

- Papaya pulp: 2 tablespoons
- Mango pulp: 2 tablespoons
- Water: a little bit

OOOOOOOOOOOOOOOOOO

Procedure:

A. Start by extracting the pulp from the papaya and mango. Scoop out the flesh of the fruits and mash them to create a smooth pulp. You will need 2 tablespoons of papaya pulp and 2 tablespoons of mango pulp.

B. In a bowl, combine the papaya pulp, mango pulp, and a small amount of water. Mix them well until you achieve a smooth consistency. The combination of papaya and mango is beneficial for your skin as they contain enzymes and antioxidants that can help reduce blackheads and promote a healthy complexion.

C. Before applying the mask, ensure that your face is clean and free from any makeup or impurities. Use a gentle cleanser or face wash to cleanse your skin thoroughly.

D. Using clean fingers or a brush, apply the mask evenly onto your face, focusing on areas with blackheads or areas that require extra attention. Allow the mask to sit on your skin for approximately 15 minutes. During this time, the nutrients from the papaya and mango will work to exfoliate and nourish your skin.

E. After 15 minutes, rinse your face with lukewarm water to remove the mask. Gently massage your skin in circular motions while rinsing to further exfoliate and promote blood circulation.

Notes:

A. Ensure that the papaya and mango are ripe for optimal results. Ripe fruits are softer and easier to extract pulp from.

B. If the consistency of the mask is too thick, you can add a little more water to achieve a spreadable consistency. Adjust the amount of water according to your preference.

C. While applying the mask, you can take this time to relax and pamper yourself. Find a comfortable position and indulge in a soothing experience.

D. It is recommended to use this papaya and mango mask once or twice a week as part of your skincare routine. Consistency is key to achieving desired results.

E. If you have sensitive skin or are prone to allergies, it is advisable to perform a patch test on a small area of your skin before applying the mask to your entire face.

F. Remember to moisturize your skin after rinsing off the mask to maintain hydration and protect your skin barrier.

G. In addition to using this homemade mask, it is important to maintain a healthy lifestyle, including a balanced diet, regular exercise, and proper skincare habits, to achieve and maintain healthy skin.

H. If you experience any adverse reactions or discomfort while using this mask, discontinue use and consult a dermatologist.

I. Results may vary depending on individual skin type and condition. Listen to your skin and adjust the frequency and ingredients of your skincare routine accordingly.

J. Enjoy the natural goodness of papaya and mango in this homemade mask, and savor the refreshing aroma and texture they provide for a luxurious skincare experience.

18. Oatmeal and Butter Mask

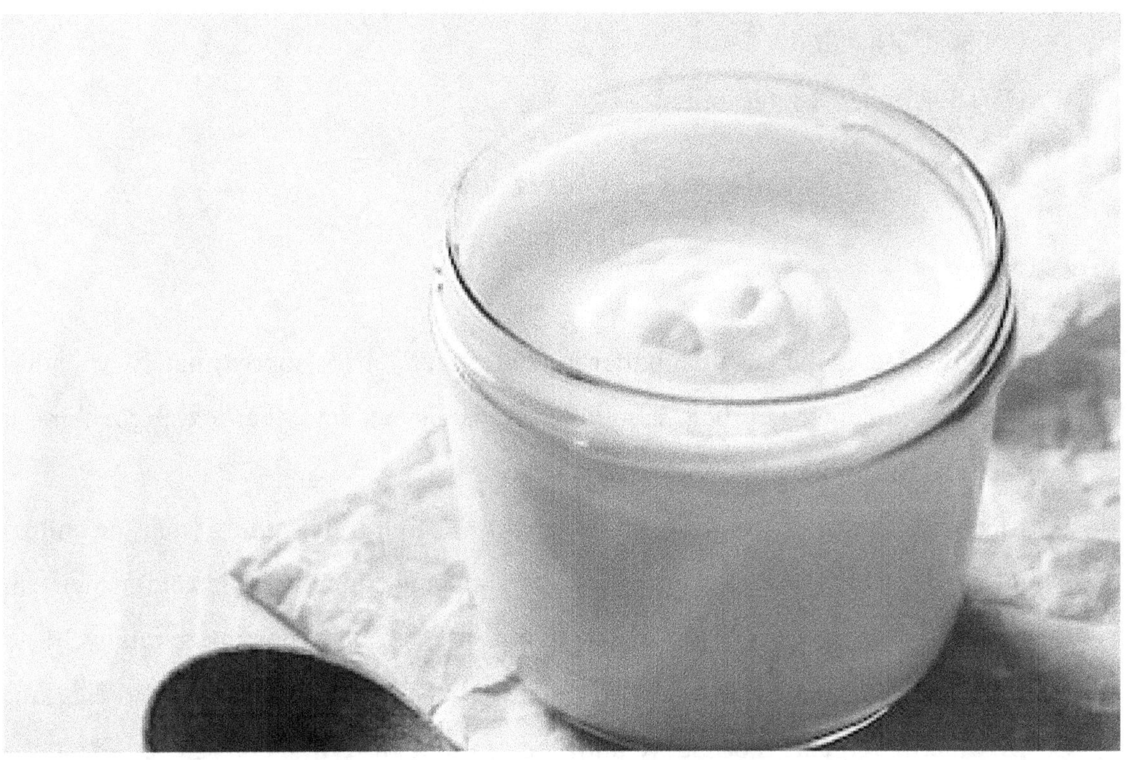

Get vitamins for your skin with oatmeal, yogurt, and butter.

Cooking Time: 5 minutes

Application Time: 15 minutes

List of Ingredients:

- Yogurt: 1 tablespoon
- Oatmeal: 1 handful
- Unsalted butter: 1 tablespoon

ooooooooooooooooo

Procedure:

A. Start by placing the unsalted butter in the refrigerator for approximately one hour. Chilling the butter will help it solidify and achieve a smoother texture, making it easier to incorporate into the mask.

B. In a bowl, combine 1 tablespoon of yogurt, 1 handful of oatmeal, and the chilled unsalted butter. The yogurt provides hydration and contains lactic acid, which can help exfoliate the skin. Oatmeal acts as a gentle exfoliant, helping to remove dead skin cells and unclog pores. The butter adds moisture and nourishment to the skin.

C. Mix the ingredients thoroughly until they form a paste-like consistency. You can use a fork or a small whisk to ensure all the ingredients are well combined. Adjust the amount of yogurt or oatmeal if needed to achieve a spreadable texture.

D. Apply the mask evenly to your face, ensuring to cover areas with blackheads or areas that require extra attention. Allow the mask to sit on your skin for approximately 15 minutes. During this time, the ingredients will work together to cleanse, exfoliate, and nourish your skin.

E. After 15 minutes, rinse your face with lukewarm water to remove the mask. Gently massage your skin while rinsing to further exfoliate and promote blood circulation. Pat your face dry with a clean towel.

Notes:

A. Make sure to use unsalted butter for this recipe. Salted butter may contain additional ingredients that can irritate the skin.

B. If you prefer a smoother mask texture, you can blend the ingredients using a blender or food processor. This will help break down the oatmeal and create a smoother consistency.

C. Feel free to adjust the quantities of the ingredients based on your preferences and the needs of your skin. If you find the mask too thick, you can add a small amount of water or more yogurt to achieve a spreadable consistency.

D. Before applying the mask, cleanse your face thoroughly to remove any dirt, oil, or makeup. This will ensure that the mask can penetrate the skin more effectively.

E. While the mask is on, you can take this time to relax and pamper yourself. Find a comfortable position and enjoy some quiet time.

F. It is recommended to use this oatmeal and butter mask once or twice a week as part of your skincare routine. Consistency is key to achieving desired results.

G. After rinsing off the mask, follow up with your regular skincare routine. Moisturize your skin to lock in hydration and protect your skin barrier.

H. If you have sensitive skin or are prone to allergies, it is advisable to perform a patch test on a small area of your skin before applying the mask to your entire face.

I. If you experience any irritation or discomfort while using this mask, discontinue use and consult a dermatologist.

J. Remember that natural ingredients may vary in potency and effectiveness, and results may vary depending on individual skin type and condition.

K. Enjoy the soothing and nourishing benefits of this homemade oatmeal and butter mask, and embrace the natural goodness it provides for your skin.

19. Egg Yolk, Honey, and Peach Mask

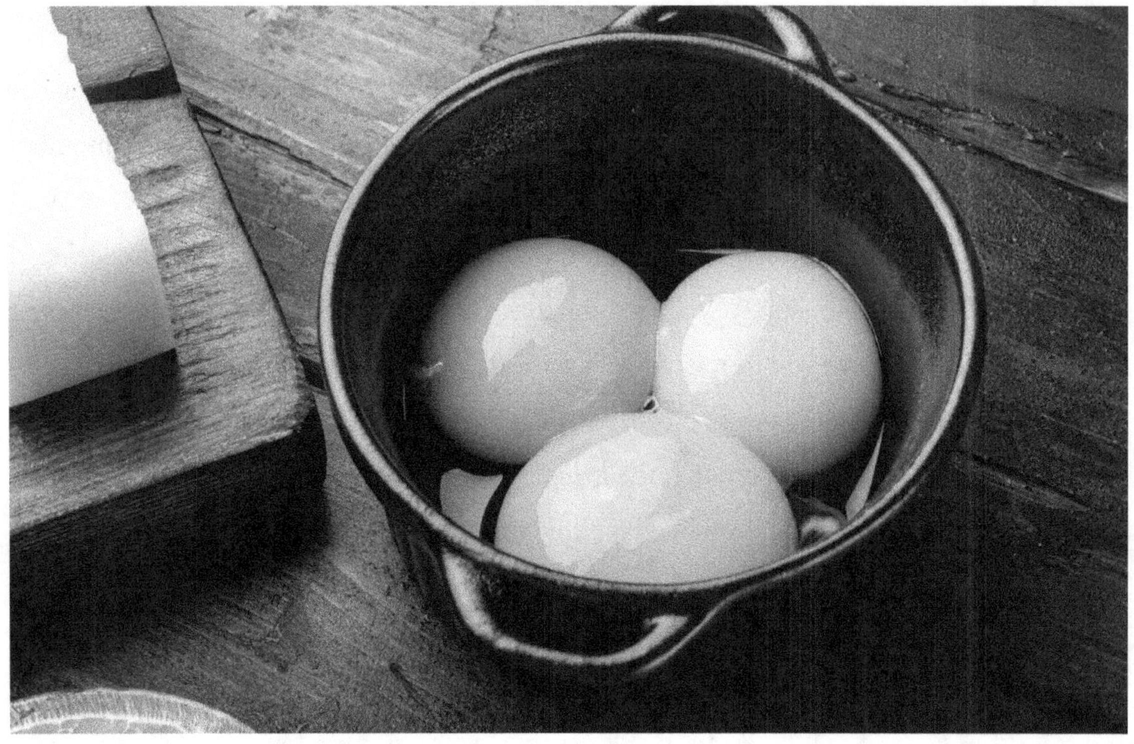

This mask is really good to moisturize your skin.

Cooking Time: 5 minutes

Application Time: 30 minutes

List of Ingredients:

- Egg yolk: 1
- Ripe peach: 1
- Honey: 1 teaspoon

OOOOOOOOOOOOOOOOOO

Procedure:

A. Start by cutting a ripe peach into small pieces. Place the peach pieces in a blender or food processor. Add 1 teaspoon of honey and 1 egg yolk to the blender as well. The peach provides antioxidants and vitamins to the skin, while honey adds hydration and antibacterial properties. The egg yolk contains proteins and nutrients that can help nourish the skin.

B. Blend the ingredients together until you achieve a smooth and creamy consistency. Make sure all the ingredients are well combined to create a uniform mixture. You can adjust the amount of honey or peach depending on your desired texture and the needs of your skin.

C. Apply the mask onto your cleansed face, ensuring to cover areas with blackheads or areas that require extra attention. Use your fingertips or a clean brush to spread an even layer of the mask over your skin. Avoid the eye and mouth areas.

D. Allow the mask to sit on your skin for approximately 25 to 30 minutes. During this time, the ingredients will work to nourish, hydrate, and soften your skin. You can relax and unwind during this period, allowing the mask to work its magic.

E. After the recommended application time has passed, rinse your face thoroughly with warm water to remove the mask. Gently massage your skin while rinsing to enhance the exfoliating effect and promote circulation. Pat your face dry with a clean towel.

Notes:

A. Make sure to use a ripe peach for this recipe as it will be easier to blend and provide more nutrients to the mask.

B. It's important to use the yolk only and discard the egg white. The egg yolk contains more nourishing properties for the skin.

C. If you have sensitive skin or are allergic to any of the ingredients, it's recommended to perform a patch test before applying the mask to your entire face.

D. Prior to applying the mask, cleanse your face thoroughly to remove any dirt, oil, or makeup. This will ensure that the mask can penetrate the skin effectively.

E. When applying the mask, be gentle and avoid rubbing or pulling on the skin, especially around delicate areas such as the eyes.

F. It's advised to use this mask once or twice a week as part of your skincare routine. Consistency is key to achieving desired results.

G. After rinsing off the mask, follow up with your regular skincare routine. Apply a moisturizer to lock in hydration and protect your skin barrier.

H. Remember that natural ingredients may vary in potency and effectiveness, and results may vary depending on individual skin type and condition.

I. If you experience any irritation or discomfort while using this mask, discontinue use and consult a dermatologist.

J. Enjoy the nourishing and refreshing benefits of this homemade egg yolk, honey, and peach mask, and embrace the natural goodness it provides for your skin.

Natural Remedies to Moisturize Winter Skin

Natural Remedies for Dry Skin

OOOOOOOOOOOOOOOOO

20. Sage and Chamomile Treatment

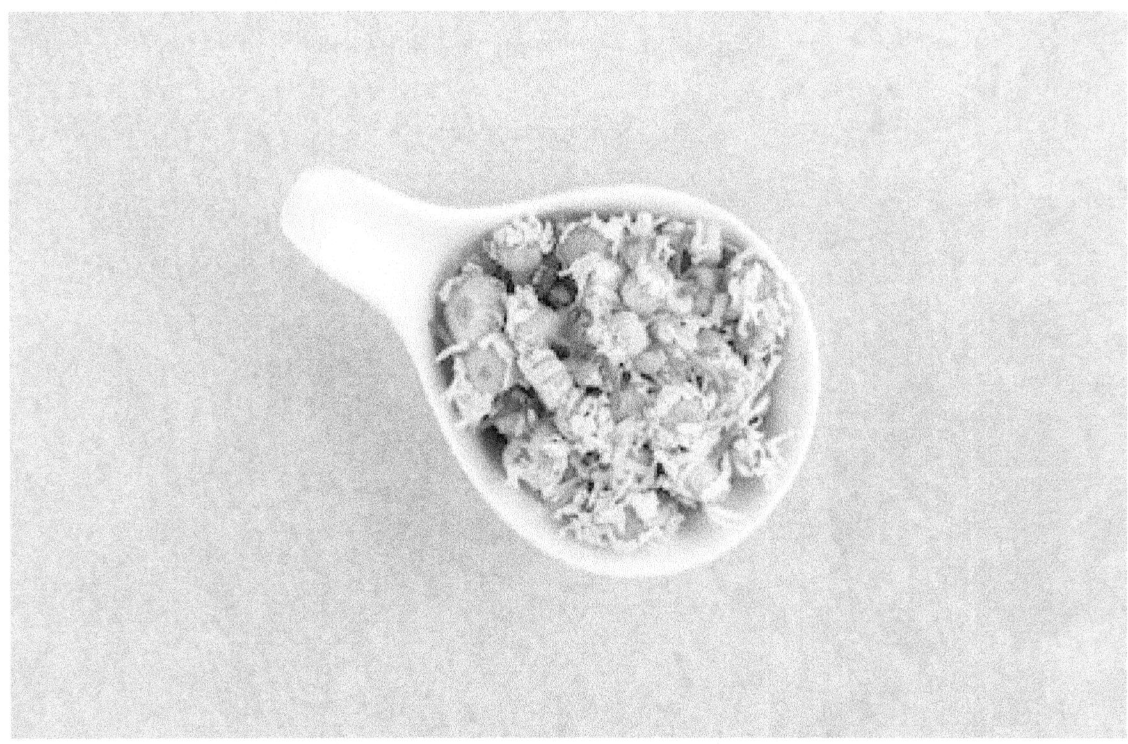

Chamomile and sage are great herbs for skin treatments.

Cooking Time: 5 minutes

Application Time: 20 minutes

List of Ingredients:

- Hot water: 2 cups
- Ground sage: 1 tablespoon
- Chamomile infusion: 3 cups

OOOOOOOOOOOOOOOOOO

Procedure:

A. Begin by boiling 3 cups of water in a pot. Once the water reaches a boil, add chamomile leaves to create a chamomile infusion. Chamomile is known for its soothing properties, which can help calm and nourish dry skin. Allow the chamomile to steep in the hot water for a few minutes to release its beneficial compounds.

B. After the chamomile infusion has steeped, add 1 tablespoon of ground sage to the pot. Sage is a natural herb that has anti-inflammatory and antioxidant properties, making it beneficial for dry skin. Stir the mixture well to combine the sage with the chamomile infusion.

C. Once the sage and chamomile infusion is well-mixed, allow the mixture to cool down slightly. You want it to be warm but comfortable to apply on your skin. Take a cotton pad or cotton bud and dip it into the mixture.

D. Gently apply the sage and chamomile mixture to your skin, focusing on areas that are dry or in need of hydration. Leave the mixture on your skin for approximately 25 minutes to allow the ingredients to penetrate and provide their nourishing benefits. After the recommended application time, rinse your skin with warm water to remove the mixture.

Notes:

A. Make sure to use hot water to create the chamomile infusion, as this will help extract the beneficial compounds from the chamomile leaves.

B. Ground sage can be found in most grocery stores or health food stores. If you have fresh sage leaves, you can grind them using a mortar and pestle or a coffee grinder to create the ground sage.

C. When applying the mixture to your skin, be gentle and avoid rubbing or pulling on the skin, especially if you have dry or sensitive skin.

D. After rinsing off the mixture, you can follow up with a moisturizer suitable for dry skin to lock in hydration and further nourish your skin.

E. It is recommended to repeat this remedy twice a week to see visible results. Consistency is key in maintaining healthy and hydrated skin.

F. If you experience any irritation or discomfort while using this treatment, discontinue use and consult a dermatologist.

G. It's important to note that individual results may vary, and it's always a good idea to consult with a dermatologist or skin care professional if you have specific concerns or persistent skin issues.

H. Enjoy the soothing and hydrating benefits of this natural sage and chamomile treatment for dry skin, and embrace the nourishing properties of these herbal ingredients.

21. Carrot Juice and Cottage Cheese

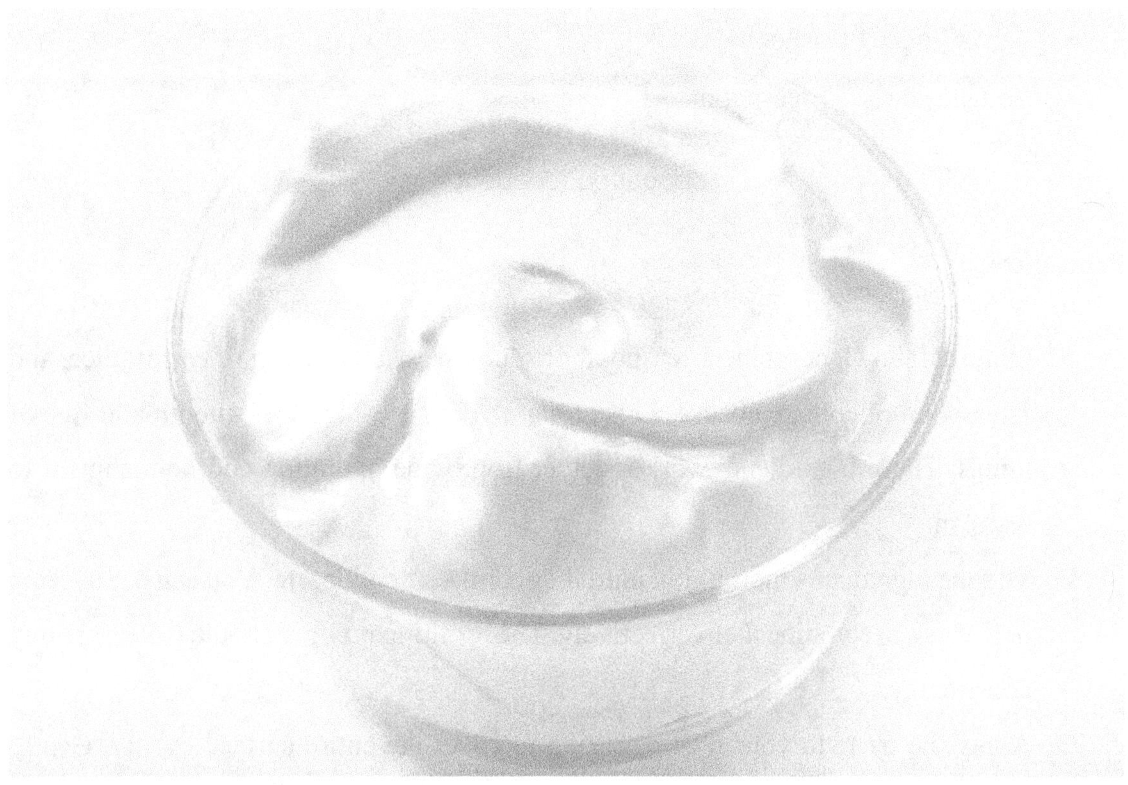

Sour cream, Cottage cheese, and organic carrot juice could treat your flaky skin magically, so put your efforts into mixing all of them.

Cooking Time: 5 minutes

Application Time: 15 minutes

List of Ingredients:

- Sour cream: 1 teaspoon
- Carrot juice: 1 teaspoon
- Cottage cheese: 1 teaspoon

OOOOOOOOOOOOOOOOOO

Procedure:

A. In a small bowl, combine 1 teaspoon of sour cream, 1 teaspoon of carrot juice, and 1 teaspoon of cottage cheese. Ensure that the cottage cheese is smooth and free of lumps. These ingredients work together to provide hydration and nourishment to dry skin.

B. Mix the ingredients thoroughly until they form a smooth paste. You can use a spoon or a whisk to combine them effectively. The resulting mixture should have a creamy consistency.

C. Apply the paste to your face, ensuring to cover the entire surface evenly. Gently massage the mixture onto your skin using circular motions. This will help the nutrients penetrate into the deeper layers of your skin for maximum benefits.

D. Allow the paste to sit on your face for approximately 15 minutes. During this time, the ingredients will work their magic, hydrating and nourishing your dry skin. After the recommended time has passed, rinse your face thoroughly with lukewarm water to remove the paste.

Notes:

A. Ensure that the cottage cheese is smooth and free of lumps before combining it with the other ingredients. This will help create a smooth and consistent paste for easier application.

B. Organic carrot juice is preferred for this recipe, as it is free from added chemicals or preservatives. However, if organic carrot juice is not available, you can use freshly squeezed carrot juice or a high-quality store-bought option.

C. When applying the paste to your face, you can use your fingers or a clean brush to spread it evenly. Be gentle and avoid tugging or pulling on your skin, especially if you have dry or sensitive skin.

D. It is recommended to leave the paste on for 15 minutes to allow the ingredients to deeply moisturize and nourish your skin. You can use this time to relax and enjoy a rejuvenating skincare routine.

E. After rinsing off the paste, gently pat your face dry with a clean towel. Follow up with a moisturizer suitable for dry skin to lock in the hydration and further nourish your skin.

F. For optimal results, it is recommended to repeat this remedy at least twice a week. Consistency is key in maintaining healthy and hydrated skin.

G. If you experience any irritation or discomfort while using this treatment, discontinue use and consult a dermatologist.

H. Remember, individual results may vary, and it's always a good idea to consult with a dermatologist or skin care professional if you have specific concerns or persistent skin issues.

I. Enjoy the hydrating and nourishing benefits of this natural carrot juice and cottage cheese remedy for dry skin, and embrace the rejuvenating properties of these ingredients.

22. Oatmeal, Lemon Peel, and Almond Treatment

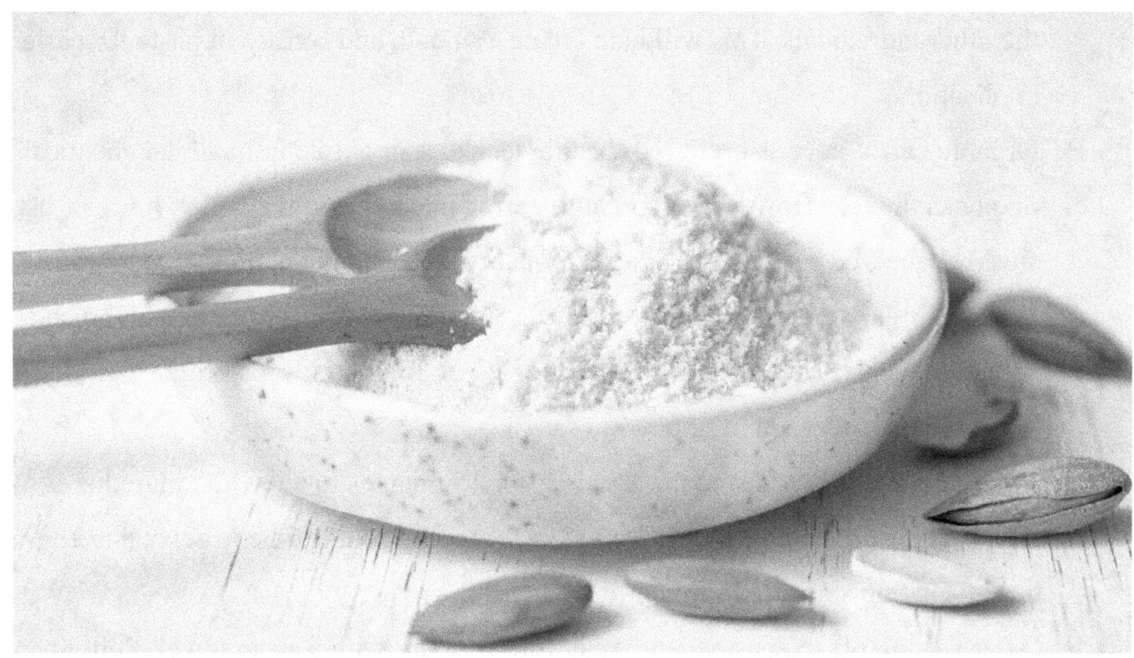

Dry sports are no more now because oatmeal, lemon peel, and almond powder which are here for your treatment.

Cooking Time: 5 minutes

Application Time: 10 to 20 minutes

List of Ingredients:

- Lemon rind: 2 teaspoons
- Oatmeal: 2 teaspoons
- Almond powder: 2 teaspoons

OOOOOOOOOOOOOOOOOO

Procedure:

A. In a bowl, combine 2 teaspoons of lemon rind, 2 teaspoons of oatmeal, and 2 teaspoons of almond powder. These ingredients work synergistically to provide gentle exfoliation and nourishment to dry skin.

B. Mix the ingredients well, ensuring they are evenly combined. You can use a spoon or your fingers to blend them together. If the mixture is too dry, you can add a small amount of pure water to achieve a paste-like consistency.

C. Apply the mixture onto your facial skin, gently massaging it in circular motions. Focus on areas that require extra attention or are prone to dryness. The oatmeal and almond powder will help exfoliate dead skin cells, while the lemon rind provides a brightening effect. Allow the mixture to dry thoroughly on your skin.

D. Once the mixture has dried completely, rinse your face with lukewarm water. Use gentle circular motions to remove the mixture, ensuring all residue is washed away. Pat your skin dry with a clean towel.

Notes:

A. When using lemon rind, ensure that you only use the outer yellow part and avoid the white pith underneath, as it can be bitter.

B. If you have sensitive skin, it is advisable to perform a patch test before applying the mixture to your entire face. Apply a small amount on the inside of your wrist or behind your ear and wait for 24 hours to check for any adverse reactions.

C. The mixture can be slightly abrasive due to the oatmeal and almond powder, so be gentle when massaging it onto your skin. Avoid applying excessive pressure, especially if you have sensitive or delicate skin.

D. It is recommended to let the mixture dry thoroughly on your face to allow the ingredients to work their magic. You can use this time to relax and enjoy a pampering skincare routine.

E. After rinsing off the mixture, gently pat your face dry with a clean towel. Follow up with a moisturizer suitable for dry skin to lock in hydration and further nourish your skin.

F. For optimal results, you can use this treatment 1-2 times a week, depending on your skin's needs. Adjust the frequency based on your skin's sensitivity and tolerance to exfoliation.

G. Remember, individual results may vary, and it's always a good idea to consult with a dermatologist or skin care professional if you have specific concerns or persistent skin issues.

H. Embrace the benefits of this natural oatmeal, lemon peel, and almond treatment for dry skin, and enjoy the rejuvenating properties of these ingredients.

23. Carrot Facial Treatment

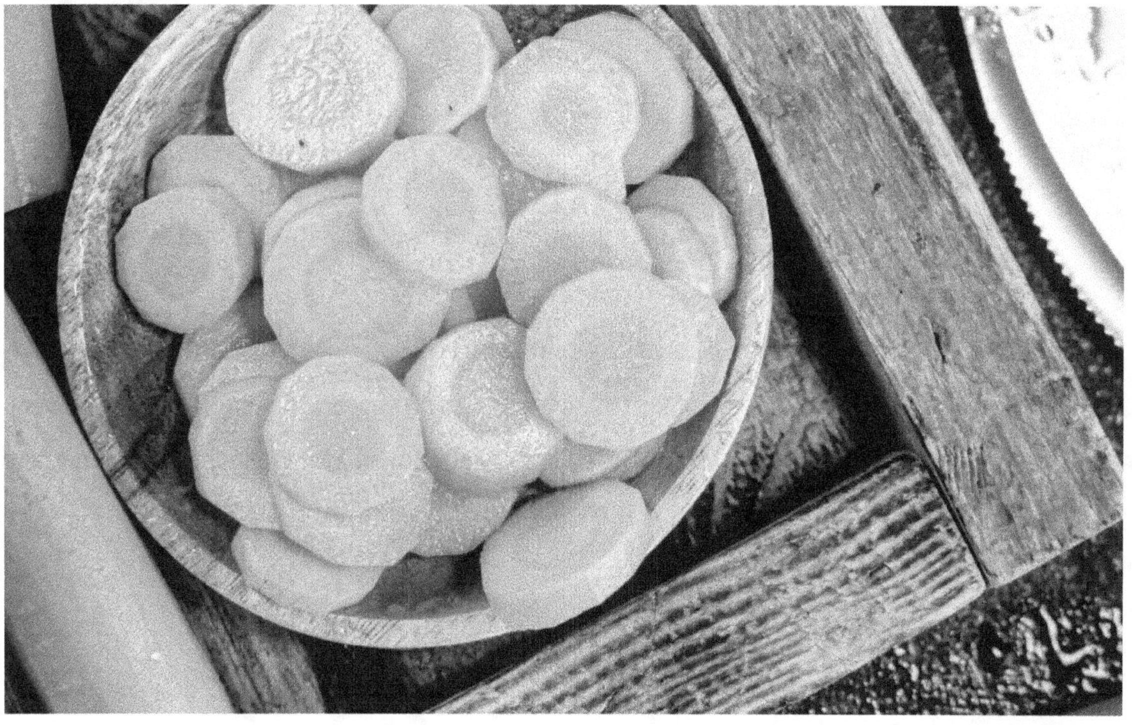

This is a very simple treatment that will help in reducing dead cells from your skin.

Cooking Time: 5 minutes

Application Time: 10 minutes

List of Ingredients:

- Carrots: 2 - 3

OOOOOOOOOOOOOOOOOO

Procedure:

A. Begin by boiling 2-3 carrots until they are tender and soft. This will help soften the carrots and make them easier to mash into a paste.

B. Once the carrots are cooked, remove them from the boiling water and allow them to cool slightly. Using a fork or a blender, mash the carrots until you achieve a smooth paste-like consistency. The natural moisture and nutrients present in carrots are beneficial for dry skin.

C. Apply the carrot paste onto your facial skin, spreading it evenly and making sure to cover all areas. Gently massage the paste into your skin using circular motions. This will help promote better absorption and circulation. Allow the carrot paste to sit on your skin for approximately 10 minutes.

D. After 10 minutes, rinse off the carrot paste with lukewarm water. Use your hands or a clean washcloth to gently remove the paste from your face. Pat your skin dry with a clean towel. The carrots' natural properties can help hydrate and nourish your dry skin, leaving it feeling refreshed and revitalized.

Notes:

A. It's important to use fresh, organic carrots for this recipe, as they contain higher levels of nutrients and are free from harmful chemicals.

B. Be cautious when handling hot carrots to avoid burning yourself. Allow them to cool slightly before mashing them into a paste.

C. For a smoother paste, you can use a blender or food processor to process the boiled carrots.

D. If desired, you can add a teaspoon of honey or a few drops of almond oil to the carrot paste for added hydration and nourishment.

E. To enhance the relaxation and soothing effects of this treatment, consider applying the carrot paste while lying down and enjoying some quiet time.

F. After rinsing off the carrot paste, follow up with a moisturizer suitable for dry skin to lock in the hydration and further nourish your skin.

G. You can incorporate this carrot facial treatment into your skincare routine once or twice a week, depending on your skin's needs and sensitivity.

H. Individual results may vary, and it's always a good idea to consult with a dermatologist or skin care professional if you have specific concerns or persistent skin issues.

24. Vodka, Honey, and Olive Oil

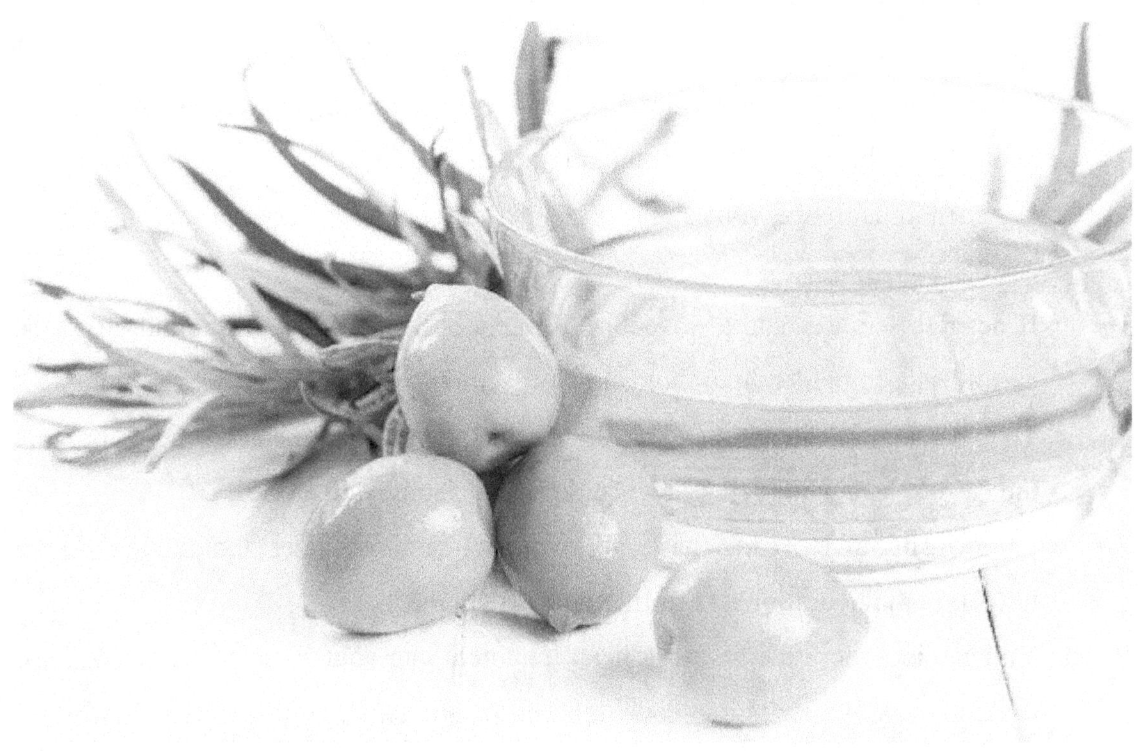

Cooking Time: 5 minutes

Application Time: 10 minutes

List of Ingredients:

- Honey: 1 tablespoon
- Olive oil: 1 tablespoon
- Vodka: 2 tablespoons

oooooooooooooooooo

Procedure:

A. In a bowl, combine 2 tablespoons of vodka, 1 tablespoon of honey, and 1 tablespoon of olive oil. Mix these ingredients well to create a smooth and consistent mixture. The combination of vodka, honey, and olive oil provides nourishment and hydration to dry skin.

B. Using a brush or your fingertips, apply the mixture onto your skin, making sure to cover all areas. Gently massage the mixture into your skin using circular motions. This helps the ingredients penetrate into the skin and enhances their effectiveness.

C. Allow the mixture to sit on your skin for approximately 10 minutes. During this time, the honey, olive oil, and vodka work together to moisturize and rejuvenate your dry skin. You may feel a slight tingling sensation from the vodka, which is normal.

D. After 10 minutes, rinse off the mixture from your skin with lukewarm water. Ensure that all traces of the mixture are removed from your face. Pat your skin dry with a clean towel. The combination of vodka, honey, and olive oil helps to hydrate and nourish dry skin, leaving it feeling soft and supple.

Notes:

A. Choose high-quality ingredients, such as raw honey and extra virgin olive oil, to maximize the benefits for your skin.

B. If you have sensitive skin, perform a patch test before applying the mixture to your entire face. Apply a small amount of the mixture on a small area of your skin and wait for 24 hours to check for any adverse reactions.

C. Use a clean brush or your fingertips to apply the mixture to avoid introducing bacteria or impurities onto your skin.

D. Remember to avoid contact with your eyes while applying the mixture.

E. For added relaxation, consider applying the mixture while lying down and enjoying a quiet moment.

F. After rinsing off the mixture, follow up with a gentle moisturizer suitable for your skin type to seal in the hydration and nourishment.

G. You can incorporate this natural remedy into your skincare routine once or twice a week, depending on the needs of your skin.

H. Individual results may vary, and it's always a good idea to consult with a dermatologist or skin care professional if you have specific concerns or persistent skin issues.

Natural Remedies for Nails and Hair

OOOOOOOOOOOOOOOOO

25. Get Shiny Hair with Banana

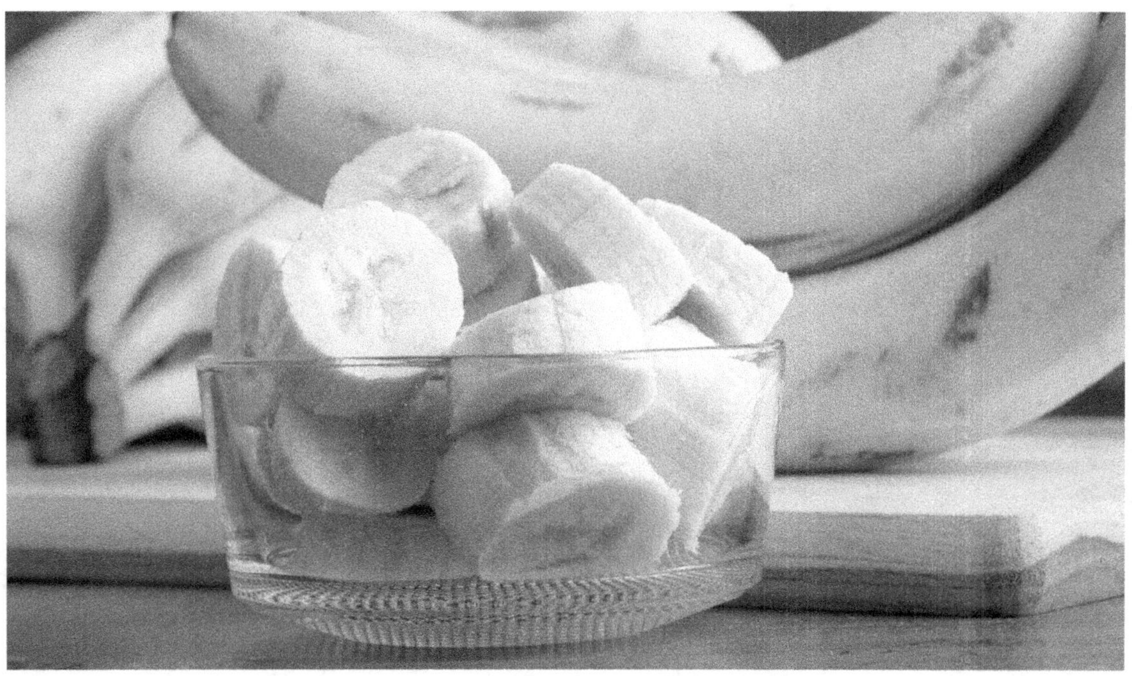

Cooking Time: 5 minutes

Application Time: 20 minutes

List of Ingredients:

- Banana: 1

ooooooooooooooooooo

Procedure:

A. Start by peeling a ripe banana and placing it in a bowl. Mash the banana with a fork or use a blender to create a smooth paste. Bananas are rich in nutrients that can nourish and hydrate your hair, promoting shine and strength.

B. Apply the mashed banana paste to your hair, making sure to cover all strands from roots to ends. You can use your fingers or a hairbrush to evenly distribute the paste. Gently massage the paste into your scalp to stimulate blood circulation and promote healthy hair growth.

C. Leave the banana paste on your hair for approximately 20 minutes. During this time, the nutrients in the banana will penetrate your hair shafts, providing deep conditioning and moisturization. You can cover your hair with a shower cap or towel to prevent the paste from dripping.

D. After 20 minutes, rinse your hair thoroughly with lukewarm water. Make sure to remove all traces of the banana paste from your hair. Follow up with a gentle shampoo to cleanse your hair and remove any residue. Finish with a conditioner to further moisturize and soften your hair.

Notes:

A. Use a ripe banana for this treatment, as it will be easier to mash into a smooth paste and will contain higher concentrations of beneficial nutrients.

B. If you have longer hair, you may need to adjust the quantity of the banana accordingly to ensure full coverage.

C. While applying the banana paste, be mindful of the potential for staining. Consider wearing an old shirt or placing a towel around your shoulders to protect your clothing.

D. Massage the banana paste into your scalp to promote scalp health and stimulate hair follicles. This can help with hair growth and overall hair health.

E. Rinse your hair thoroughly to remove all traces of the banana paste. Residue left in the hair can cause stickiness or an unpleasant smell when dry.

F. Follow up with your regular hair care routine after the treatment, including using a conditioner to keep your hair hydrated and manageable.

G. This banana natural remedy can be used once a week or as needed to provide shine and nourishment to your hair.

26. Get Strong Nails with Garlic

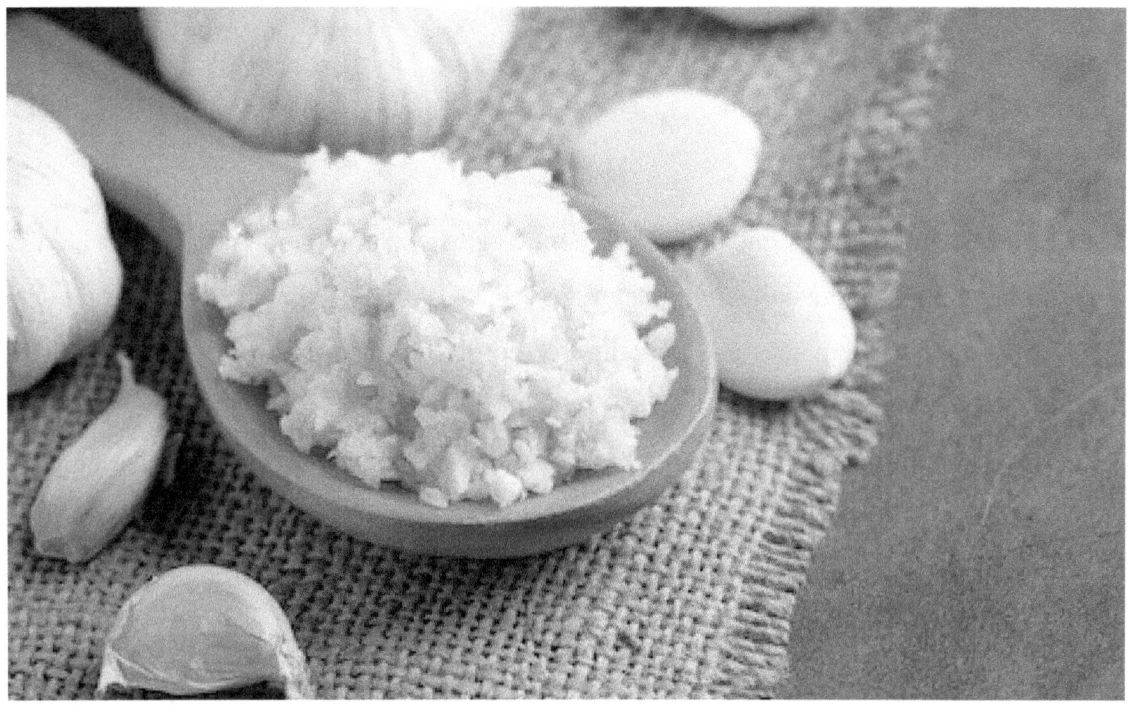

Cooking Time: 5 minutes

Application Time: 10 minutes

List of Ingredients:

- Chopped garlic: a few pieces

ooooooooooooooooooo

Procedure:

A. Start by gathering a few pieces of chopped garlic. Garlic contains sulfur, which is known to promote nail strength and growth.

B. Place the garlic pieces in a container or bottle of your preferred nail treatment or base coat. You can use a clear nail polish or a specific nail strengthening product. Make sure the container is tightly sealed to prevent evaporation and maintain the potency of the garlic.

C. Let the garlic infuse in the nail formula for at least 9 days. During this time, the beneficial compounds from the garlic will be released into the formula, enriching it with nutrients that can help strengthen your nails.

D. After the 9-day infusion period, apply the nail formula with the infused garlic on your nails as you would with regular nail polish. Use a brush to evenly distribute the formula over your nails. Allow it to dry completely before applying additional layers or nail polish colors, if desired.

Notes:

A. The garlic infusion process allows the beneficial compounds from garlic to transfer into the nail formula, promoting stronger and healthier nails.

B. Choose a nail treatment or base coat that you regularly use, as this will ensure that you incorporate the garlic infusion into your nail care routine.

C. It's important to store the garlic-infused nail formula in a cool and dark place, away from direct sunlight, to preserve its potency.

D. When applying the garlic-infused nail formula, ensure that it covers the entire nail surface, including the tips and cuticles, for maximum benefit.

E. The length of time you keep the garlic-infused formula on your nails can vary. You can choose to remove it before applying colored nail polish or keep it on for an extended period as a nail treatment.

F. It's normal to experience a slight garlic scent while using this natural remedy. If the odor is bothersome, you can try using scented hand creams or oils after removing the garlic-infused formula.

G. Consistency is key. Apply the garlic-infused nail formula regularly to see noticeable improvements in nail strength over time.

H. If you experience any irritation or discomfort, discontinue use and consult a dermatologist.

27. Natural Conditioner for Swimming

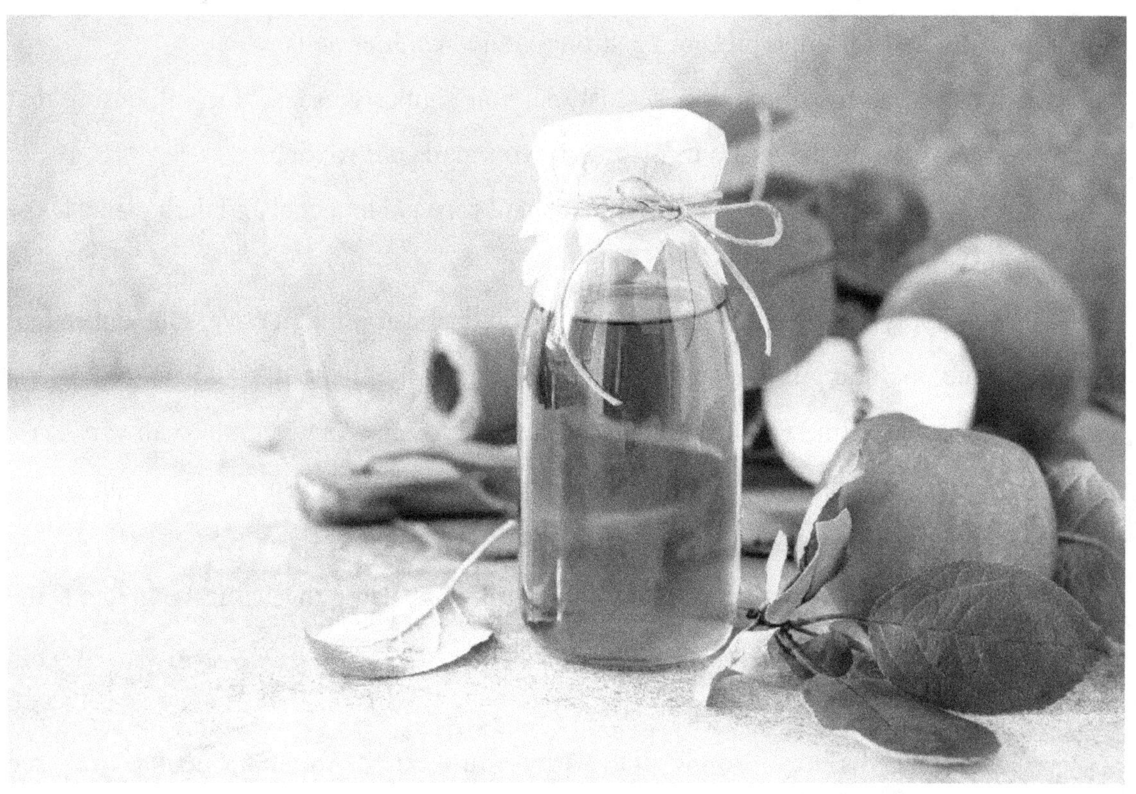

If you want to protect your water from chlorine, try this blend before swimming or even going out for a beach day.

Cooking Time: 5 minutes

Application Time: Until swimming

List of Ingredients:

- Water: ¾ cup
- Apple cider vinegar: ¼ cup

OOOOOOOOOOOOOOOOOO

Procedure:

A. Start by combining ¾ cup of water and ¼ cup of apple cider vinegar. Apple cider vinegar is known for its ability to remove chlorine and mineral buildup from hair, making it a great natural conditioner for swimmers.

B. Transfer the mixture into a spray bottle. This will allow for easy application and distribution of the conditioner throughout your hair.

C. Spray the mixture onto your hair, focusing on the roots and working your way down to the tips. The roots are particularly susceptible to chlorine and mineral buildup, so it's important to apply the blend there for maximum protection.

D. Gently comb through your hair to ensure that the conditioner is evenly distributed. Leave the conditioner in your hair for a few minutes to allow it to work its magic, and then rinse thoroughly with water.

Notes:

A. This natural conditioner is specifically designed to counteract the effects of chlorine and mineral buildup that can occur from swimming in pools.

B. Apple cider vinegar helps to restore the pH balance of your hair and remove any residue left by chlorine and minerals, leaving your hair feeling soft and smooth.

C. Adjust the quantities of water and apple cider vinegar depending on the length and thickness of your hair. You can increase or decrease the amounts to suit your hair's needs.

D. It's recommended to use this natural conditioner after swimming sessions to help protect your hair from damage caused by chlorine and other chemicals found in pool water.

E. For optimal results, rinse your hair thoroughly after using the natural conditioner to ensure that all traces of chlorine and vinegar are removed.

F. This natural conditioner can be used in conjunction with your regular shampoo and conditioner routine.

G. If you prefer, you can add a few drops of essential oil to the mixture to mask the smell of vinegar. Lavender, rosemary, or peppermint essential oils work well for this purpose.

H. Keep in mind that this natural conditioner is not a substitute for regular hair care. It's important to maintain a healthy hair care routine, including regular shampooing, conditioning, and trimming, to keep your hair in its best condition.

I. If you have any known allergies or sensitivities to apple cider vinegar, it's advisable to perform a patch test before using this conditioner on your entire head of hair.

J. Enjoy the benefits of this natural conditioner and protect your hair from the damaging effects of chlorine while swimming.

28. Botanical Oil for Dry and Damaged Hair

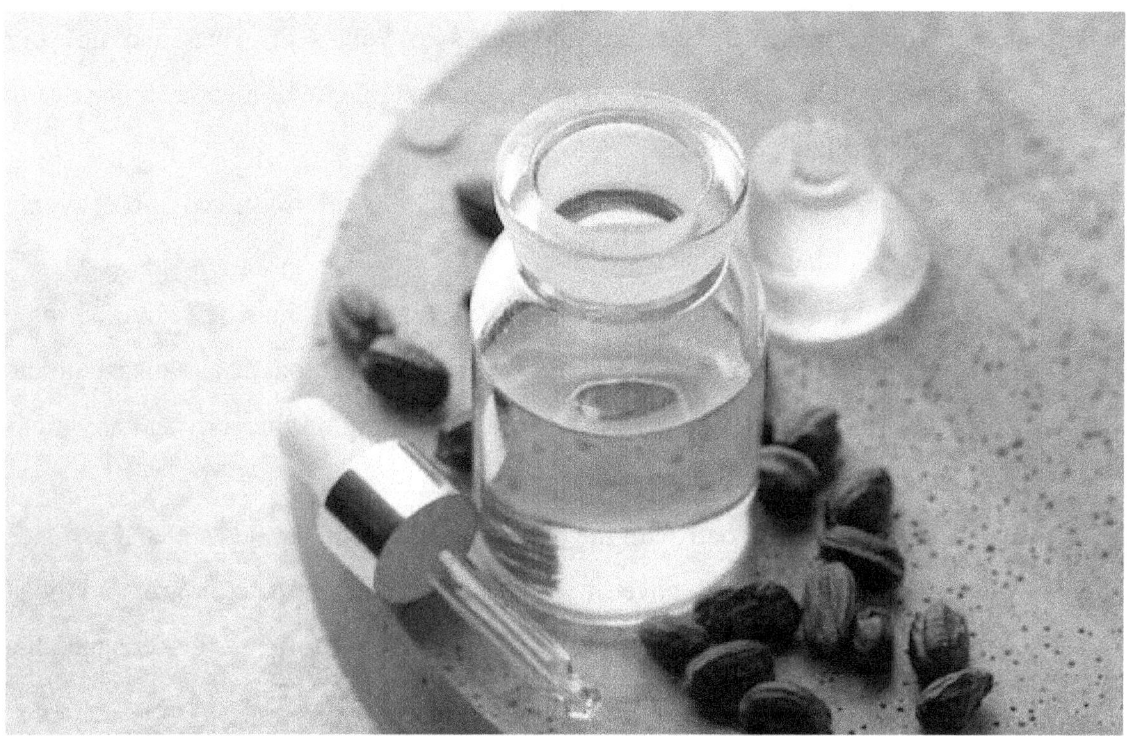

You can get the benefits of botanical oil from sweet almond oil, jojoba oil, and olive oil.

Application Time: 30 minutes

List of Ingredients:

- Botanical oil (jojoba oil, olive oil, coconut oil, and sweet almond oil): choose any one of them

OOOOOOOOOOOOOOOOOO

Procedure:

A. Choose one of the botanical oils such as jojoba oil, olive oil, coconut oil, or sweet almond oil. Consider the texture and needs of your hair when making your selection. If you have heavy and thick hair, coconut oil can be a good choice due to its deep moisturizing properties.

B. Dampen your hair with water. This will help the oil to spread more evenly throughout your hair.

C. Apply a small quantity of the chosen botanical oil to your hair. Start by pouring a few drops of oil into your palm and then rub your hands together to distribute the oil. Gently run your hands through your hair, focusing on the ends and any areas that are particularly dry or damaged.

D. Thoroughly cover your hair with the oil, ensuring that all strands are coated. Once your hair is coated with oil, cover it with a shower cap to create a warm and moist environment. Wrap a warm towel around the shower cap to further enhance the conditioning process.

E. Leave the oil in your hair for approximately 30 minutes to allow it to deeply penetrate and moisturize your strands. This period of time allows the botanical oil to work its magic and nourish your dry and damaged hair.

F. After 30 minutes, remove the shower cap and towel. Rinse your hair with warm water to remove the excess oil. It's recommended to use a natural shampoo to cleanse your hair and remove any remaining oil.

G. Pat your hair dry with a towel and style as desired. You should notice that your hair feels softer, smoother, and more hydrated after this botanical oil treatment.

Notes:

A. Botanical oils such as jojoba oil, olive oil, coconut oil, and sweet almond oil are rich in vitamins, minerals, and fatty acids that can nourish and restore dry and damaged hair.

B. When choosing the botanical oil, consider your hair's needs and characteristics. Coconut oil is especially beneficial for heavy and thick hair due to its ability to deeply moisturize.

C. It's important to dampen your hair before applying the oil to ensure even distribution and maximum absorption.

D. Use a small quantity of oil to avoid weighing down your hair. Start with a few drops and increase the amount if necessary, depending on the length and thickness of your hair.

E. The shower cap and warm towel create a warm and moist environment, allowing the oil to penetrate deeply into your hair shafts and provide intensive hydration.

F. Adjust the duration of the treatment based on your hair's condition. If your hair is severely dry and damaged, you can leave the oil in for a longer period, such as overnight, for more intensive treatment.

G. Rinse your hair with warm water to remove the excess oil. Avoid using hot water, as it can strip away the natural oils from your hair.

H. Use a natural shampoo to cleanse your hair after the treatment. This will help to remove any remaining oil and leave your hair feeling clean and refreshed.

I. It's recommended to incorporate this botanical oil treatment into your hair care routine on a weekly or bi-weekly basis, depending on your hair's needs.

J. Enjoy the benefits of this natural and nourishing treatment, and embrace healthier, more hydrated, and revitalized hair.

29. Natural Shampoo for Oily Hair

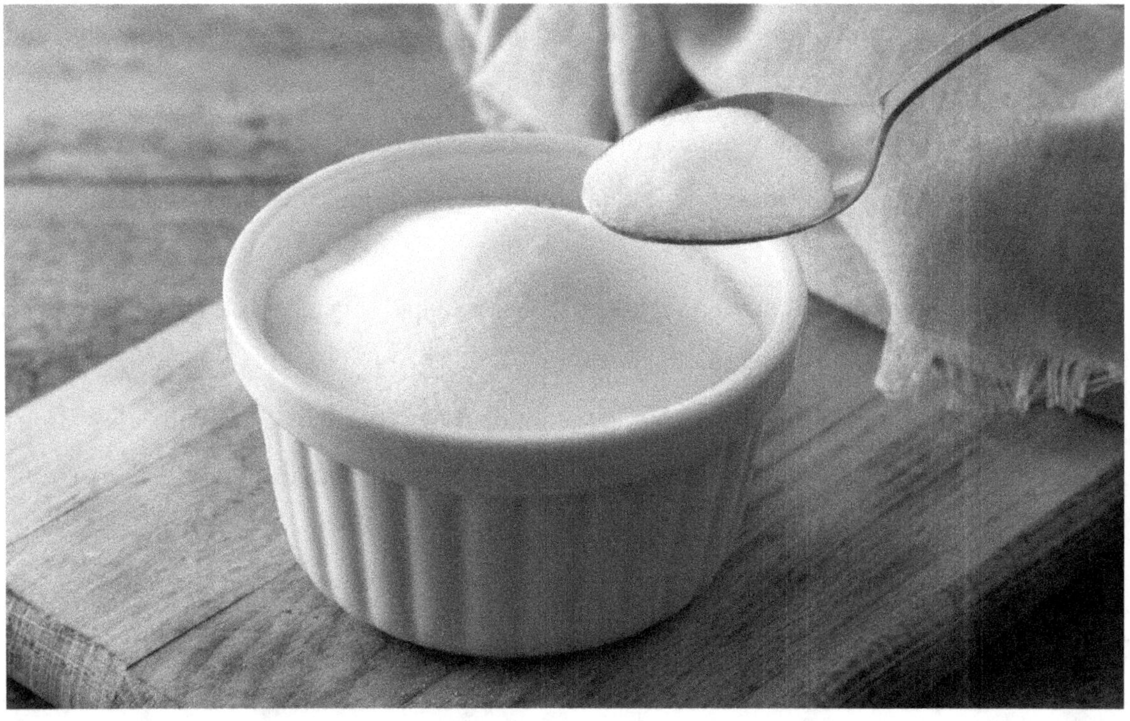

Baking soda is a good ingredient to get rid of excessive oil in your hair.

Cooking Time: 5 minutes

Application Time: 5 minutes

List of Ingredients:

- Water: 1 cup
- Baking soda: 1 tablespoon

OOOOOOOOOOOOOOOOOO

Procedure:

A. In a container, combine 1 cup of water and 1 tablespoon of baking soda. Stir the mixture well to ensure that the baking soda is dissolved in the water. Baking soda helps to cleanse the hair and scalp by removing excess oil and residue.

B. Wet your hair thoroughly with water. Make sure your hair is completely saturated before applying the natural shampoo.

C. Pour the baking soda and water mixture onto your scalp. Gently massage the liquid into your scalp using your fingertips. Focus on the roots of your hair, where oil tends to accumulate the most. Continue massaging for approximately 3 minutes to allow the baking soda to cleanse and clarify your scalp.

D. Rinse your hair thoroughly with fresh water. Ensure that all traces of the baking soda mixture are rinsed out completely.

Notes:

A. Baking soda is an effective natural ingredient for removing excess oil and buildup from the hair and scalp. It helps to balance the pH level of the scalp, reducing oiliness and promoting a cleaner, fresher feeling.

B. Ensure that your hair is fully saturated with water before applying the baking soda mixture. This helps to distribute the mixture evenly and allows for better penetration and cleansing.

C. Use your fingertips to gently massage the mixture into your scalp. Be careful not to be too harsh or vigorous, as this can potentially irritate the scalp.

D. Focus on massaging the roots of your hair, as this is where oil tends to accumulate. By targeting the scalp, you can effectively address excess oil production.

E. Massage the baking soda mixture into your scalp for approximately 3 minutes. This allows enough time for the baking soda to work its cleansing properties and absorb excess oil.

F. Rinse your hair thoroughly with fresh water to ensure that all traces of the baking soda mixture are removed. It's important to rinse your hair well to avoid any residue that may weigh down the hair or leave it feeling gritty.

G. After rinsing, you can follow up with a conditioner or natural rinse if desired. This will help to restore moisture to your hair and provide additional nourishment.

H. This natural shampoo can be used as an occasional treatment for oily hair. It helps to clarify the scalp and remove excess oil, leaving your hair feeling refreshed and less greasy.

I. It's recommended to use this natural shampoo in moderation, as baking soda can be drying if used too frequently. Once a week or every few weeks should be sufficient, depending on your hair's oiliness.

J. Adjust the amount of baking soda and water according to your hair's needs. If you have thicker or longer hair, you may need to increase the quantities accordingly.

K. Enjoy the benefits of this natural shampoo for oily hair, and embrace a cleaner, healthier scalp and refreshed locks.

30. Water and Soy Sauce Make Your Locks Shine

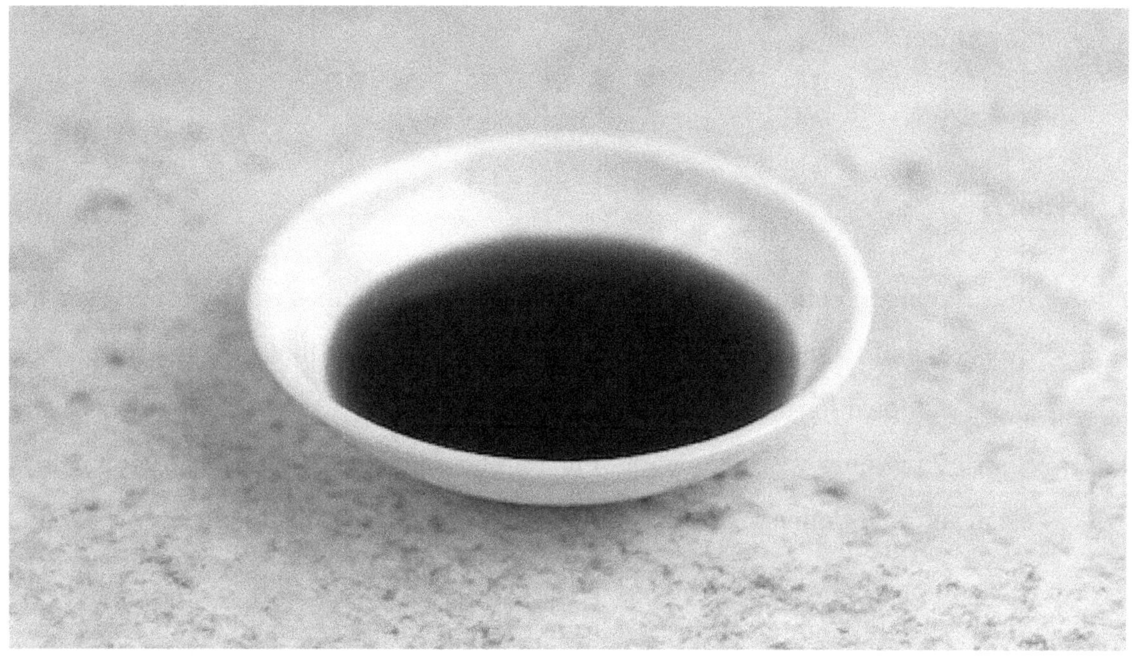

If you want to add some volume to your locks then instead of using styling gels and sprays you should try this and get great results.

Cooking Time: 5 minutes

Application Time: 15 minutes

List of Ingredients:

- Warm water: 1 cup
- Soy sauce: 1 ounce

OOOOOOOOOOOOOOOOOO

Procedure:

A. In a container, combine 1 cup of warm water and 1 ounce of soy sauce. Stir the mixture well to ensure that the soy sauce is evenly distributed in the water. Soy sauce is known for its conditioning properties that can help add shine to your hair.

B. Start by washing your hair with your regular shampoo. Ensure that your hair is clean and free from any product buildup before applying the mixture.

C. Once your hair is shampooed, apply the water and soy sauce mixture to your hair. Make sure to saturate your tresses from roots to ends, ensuring that all strands are coated with the mixture. Gently massage the mixture into your scalp and hair, paying extra attention to the ends.

D. Leave the mixture in your hair for 10 to 15 minutes. This allows the conditioning properties of the soy sauce to penetrate the hair shaft and provide nourishment and shine.

E. After the designated time has passed, rinse your hair thoroughly with lukewarm water. It's important to rinse your hair well to remove all traces of the mixture. Use your fingers or a wide-toothed comb to help distribute the water and remove the mixture completely from your locks.

F. Repeat this treatment once a week to maintain shiny and healthy locks. Consistency is key to reap the benefits of this natural remedy.

Notes:

A. Warm water and soy sauce make a simple yet effective mixture to add shine to your hair. The soy sauce contains amino acids and proteins that can help nourish and condition the hair, promoting a healthy and glossy appearance.

B. Before applying the water and soy sauce mixture, ensure that your hair is clean and free from any product buildup. This allows the mixture to penetrate the hair more effectively and deliver optimal results.

C. When applying the mixture, make sure to saturate your hair from roots to ends, ensuring that all strands are coated. Massage the mixture into your scalp to stimulate blood circulation and promote hair health.

D. Leave the mixture in your hair for 10 to 15 minutes to allow the conditioning properties of the soy sauce to work. You can use this time to relax or continue with your regular shower routine.

E. Rinse your hair thoroughly with lukewarm water after the designated time. It's crucial to remove all traces of the mixture to avoid any lingering scent or residue.

F. To help distribute the water and remove the mixture from your hair, use your fingers or a wide-toothed comb while rinsing. This helps to ensure that every strand is thoroughly rinsed and cleansed.

G. For best results, repeat this treatment once a week. Consistency is key to maintaining shiny and healthy locks over time.

H. Enjoy the benefits of this natural remedy and embrace the enhanced shine and vitality of your hair.

Conclusion

How lovely these were to assemble, and we believe they would bless your home as much as they did our hearts.

The fun part is that you can mix and match the scents on different days for varying moods. What a fun way to maximize the good feelings of the holidays.

Which scent blend do you hope to kick off with?

Author's Afterthoughts

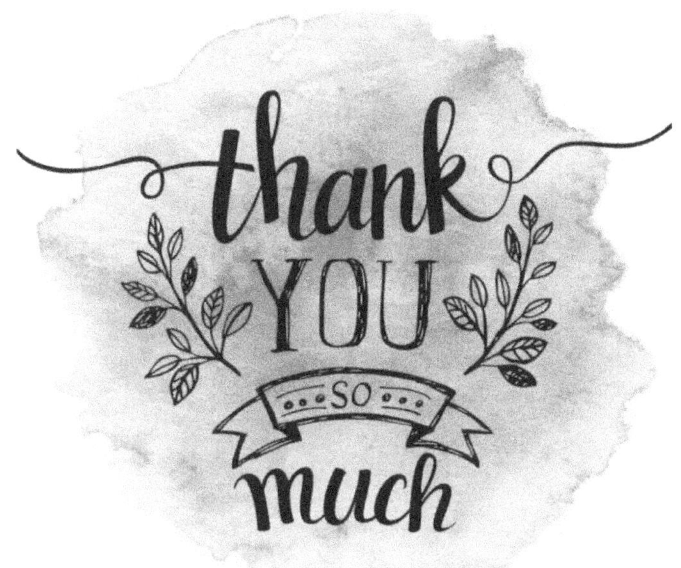

Thank you for reading my book. Your feedback is important to me. It would be greatly appreciated if you could please take a moment to REVIEW this book on Amazon so that we could make our next version better

Thanks!

Jenny Kings